Depression Confessions

Truths about Living with Depression

Victoria Mennare

Printed in the United States of America

First Printing, 2018

ISBN 9781731590503

Kindle Direct Publishing

This book is for all who live with depression and anxiety.

This book is for those who support and love someone that lives with depression or anxiety.

This book is for those who have lost someone to suicide.

This book is to break the stigma on mental illness.

This book is for me – to write my story and let it help those around me.

Contents

What is this book?

This book started as a series of Facebook and blog posts that I entitled "Depression Confessions" during the course of my most recent relapse of depression.

I am just your average, mid-twenties woman who fights Major Depressive Disorder and General Anxiety Disorder. I am also a suicide loss survivor having lost my dad to suicide in 2010. I've lived with depression since high-school, but it was not life threatening until 2015 when I was hospitalized for suicidal thoughts for the first time. I was in recovery until May, 2018 when I again became suicidal and underwent another partial hospitalization program. My recovery journey has been long and difficult – it is ongoing. This book isn't written *after* I went through depression – it's written *while* I am going through depression.

I am not a mental health professional – I'm not even a writer...I only know what I have experienced. I do not intend this book to be a self-help guide or to give advice. I only want to share my story. My story is just one of millions across the world – but if my story helps someone make sense of their own journey then I want to do that.

I also have included confessions from over 50 others that struggle with depression, have lost someone to suicide or supports someone with a mental health condition.

These confessions are meant to show people that they are not alone in their fight with mental illness. They are meant to help others understand their depression in a way that other books don't.

This project was just as much for me as it was for you, dear reader. It has helped me grow and learn about myself and my journey with depression and anxiety.

Depression

{Depression Confession #1}

I "have it all" and have depression.

I have a wonderful family, great friends, and an amazing career that I love. I have a house, my two fur babies, and a husband that loves me. In all honesty – my life is damn good.

But I have depression.

It's bad enough to be depressed when life is hard and things aren't going your way...but it's worse when everything in your life is going right. People expect you to be happy because you're doing so well in life. But the truth is - it's not that simple.

My depression isn't dependent on things going wrong in my life – because my life is actually quite great. My depression happens anyway. Even though I have everything I could ask for in life – I still battle depression. It works its way deep into my life even when things are going well.

Depression does not discriminate based on what you have in life, by your gender or age, race or ethnicity, religion or beliefs.

Depression doesn't just happen to young kids. It doesn't just happen to girls or women. It doesn't happen only to the poor or homeless.

It happens to the middle-aged man working on your car, the elderly woman walking down the street, the twelve-year-old kid playing basketball at the park, the woman who smiles at you at the grocery store checkout. It even happens to the rich and famous that, to society, literally has it all.

{Depression Confession #2}

For me, depression is feeling everything and nothing at the same time.

Depression feels like I'm drowning in emotions, yet drowning in nothingness, gasping to breathe between the waves of anguish. I feel everything and nothing at the same time.

Depression isn't always sadness and tears like it's so often perceived. It can be a number of emotions ranging from numbness and feeling nothing at all to anger, to loneliness, and fear.

For me – depression is a dark cloud of numbness and fear. Fear of feeling this way again – fear of not getting better – fear of those I love leaving me. I feel anger towards my brain for failing me. I feel hopeless – that I will feel like this forever. Sometimes I'm so overwhelmed with emotions that I can't accurately describe what I'm feeling.

I do feel happiness and excitement periodically – it's not impossible to feel happy when you have depression. (See next confession)

Depression is feeling every emotion and yet nothing at the same time. The emotion can change in a fraction of a second. Some days I feel "all" the emotions in a single day. Other days I feel absolutely nothing at all. I have to work to stay afloat above the waves of emptiness.

It's exhausting either way.

{Depression Confession #3}

I can be happy while fighting depression.

Like I said – depression can be many different emotions all at once. Happiness is one of those emotions.

It feels like looking at the happiness in my life with a film of cloudiness covering it all, but it is still there. Sometimes the sunshine can peak through and I feel genuine happiness but oftentimes it's dull and dimmed.

There are days where the depression isn't as dark and happiness is there like an old friend. Those days are few and far between but they can happen.

Just because I have depression doesn't mean I that I can't smile. I must fight to smile each day – to get out of bed – to do the things I love. Depression does not make it impossible to be happy…. but it makes it really hard sometimes.

Some might think that if I'm depressed, I can't be happy, or if I'm happy - I'm not allowed to be depressed. But I CAN be happy at times during my depression.

{Depression Confession #4}

Depression affects every aspect of my life.

Depression affects my daily activities, my job, and my relationships.

It's the simple, daily tasks like showering and getting out of bed that prove themselves difficult and sometimes nearly impossible.

I sometimes go all day without eating or go a week without showering or brushing my teeth...disgusting, I know – but when I can't even get off the couch, it's the best I can do.

I can go weeks without cleaning my house, folding laundry or doing the dishes. I want to have a clean house, but I don't have the energy.

I've had to turn to FMLA (Family Medical Leave Act) in order to keep my job but still take the time I need for appointments, therapy and mental health days. I've had to take days off of work and leave my partner to work alone in the chaos of our job at the hospital.

Relationships have suffered because I don't text back or call. I make excuses to not go somewhere or do something. It's not that I don't want to see these people – it's that it takes so much energy that I just don't have...and then all of a sudden, it's been 6 months, and then a year, and then more.

I'm not lazy – it's the fact that I can barely keep my eyes open some days, let alone interact with people or care for myself. I WANT to do these things – I do. But when my depression is at its worst – it's all I can do to get out of bed in the morning.

It touches every inch of my life.

{Depression Confession #5}

Depression turns me into someone I don't even know.

Looking in the mirror and not recognizing who I see is devastating. Sometimes I stand in front of the mirror and watch myself cry – watch the tears run down the face of someone I don't know. I want to punch the mirror out so that person doesn't exist anymore.

Sometimes I forget who I am during my depression and anxiety. I forget that I'm alive and breathing.

It's like looking into the eyes of a stranger with no hope, no love and no life. I go through the steps of someone else's life, just trying to get to the end of each day.

I used to be a go-getter, fun-loving, motivated girl who loved life and all it gave me...but in the depths of my depression, I'm far from that. I'm sad and lonely...I'm angry because I want to be different. I want to be healthy. I want to be ME.

I miss the woman I used to be.

I don't know if I'll ever be her again...It's been too long. I am a new person...with or without the depression...I have changed. But I think that the change can be good too – I'm stronger. I love fiercely and fight passionately. I have learned more about myself through the depression. I have learned that I want to live – I want to be more than a hollow vessel for my soul. I want more.

{Depression Confession #6}

My depression affects everyone around me and I am so sorry.

It affects my family, my husband, friends, and my co-workers.

I forget to text back my friends. I cancel plans last minute. I change my mind constantly or can't even make up my mind. I get irritable and take it out on my husband. I have panic attacks that ruin plans or that make me leave work.

I often feel like a burden. I'm afraid of "bringing the mood down" with my depression. I'm afraid people will leave because they don't want to be around someone so sad.

My coworkers have had to pick up my slack on days when I'm struggling at work. I'm so grateful for them.

I have lost many friends and relationships due to my depression and anxiety. Those around me didn't understand what I was going through and decided it would be easier to leave than to try to understand. I don't blame them. I'm not a fun person to be around when I'm fighting my depression.

I had to educate the people around me about depression. The ones that chose to listen and learn have now been my strongest support system.

This is what I tell them they need to know:
- I'm sorry if I cancel plans...I probably can't get myself off the couch.

- I'm sorry if I don't respond to messages or texts – I don't know what to say.
- I may get overwhelmed easily or have panic attacks randomly for no apparent reason.
- Please be patient with me. I am working so hard to get this under control.
- I will reach out to you if I need help – you don't need to walk on eggshells around me.
- ***Thank you for loving me through this.***

{Depression Confession #7}

Depression feels like I'm being bullied from the inside out.

I often feel like I have two brains. One that is logical and...well, the other is a lying, sneaky SOB. I call the one logical and the other chaos. The two fight constantly and I'm just caught in the middle. It's extremely difficult to have two pieces of yourself fighting like your life is a tug-of-war game.

My chaos brain bullies me from the inside and tells me I'm hopeless, worthless, and that I'm a failure.

The lies that my chaos brain tells me can be so overwhelming, but I know that they are lies. My logical brain tells me that I am **not** hopeless. I am **not** worthless, and I am **not** a failure.

The daily battle against my own chaos brain is exhausting. It is a constant fight against the lies my brain wants me to believe.

Example:

What happened: I wanted to clean my office, but spilled a box of art supplies.

Simple fix, right?

What my chaos brain did: "It's a mess, it's all a mess. My life is a mess! I am a mess! I can't do anything right. I'm so dumb! Just quit."

That is what a brain with depression does.

My logical brain then usually steps in after I've had my freak out or break down and tells the chaos portion to get out. The logical part of my brain reminds me that just because I spilled a box of art supplies does not mean I'm a failure or that I'm a mess. It just means I have to clean up some art supplies.

The two brains battle it out daily in my head. The chaos throwing all sorts of distorted thinking at me to make me believe its lies and the logical brain throwing back...well...logic and reality to remind me that I'm actually okay.

Many times – it can take days for the logical portion to gain back control. I've had periods of time when I feel like the logical portion of my brain is gone and I've completely "lost my mind". It truly feels like you are "going crazy". It's terrifying and like I've said...completely exhausting.

{Depression Confession #8}

Depression is NOT a choice.

I would **NEVER** choose to be this way.

I feel alone, exhausted, anxious, angry, frustrated. I feel empty. I feel hopeless and dead inside. Why would anyone choose that?

I would much rather be a functional human being who doesn't panic at the thought of leaving the house or cry for no apparent reason.

It's a no brainer that if I had the option of being happy or depressed, I would choose happiness...I think most people would. Depression is an illness not a choice just as cancer and diabetes are illnesses not choices.

I didn't choose to have depression any more than I choose to have blue eyes.

Now choosing to get help and to reach out is a choice.... it's a damn difficult one...one that is terrifying. But it can be a life changing and life-saving choice. *It saved mine.*

If you are ready to make the choice to reach out and get help – make an appointment with your primary care doctor or a psychiatrist to discuss options.

{Depression Confession #9}

Brain fog is real.

Brain fog is difficult to describe to someone who has never experienced it, but I'll do my best. It is a very disorienting experience.

It's like I'm half asleep and underwater. It's seeing the world moving in slow motion. It's seeing the world through a lens that is dirty and cracked but I'm expected to be myself and do my job/live my life as if it's perfectly clear.

It can be very difficult to form concrete thoughts. I struggle to stay focused and on task when my brain basically feels like mush.

When people ask me how I am when I have brain fog, I will most likely say I just feel a little "off" today...but in reality, I couldn't be more "off" if I tried.

It feels like my brain is only half charged and it's being forced to run at full power – but it's lagging. Like when your computer needs to buffer or your TV during a storm. That is what my brain feels like some days.

I have yet to find a way to get rid of the brain fog days. In the meantime I just do my best to stay afloat.

{Depression Confession #10}

When something bad happens – my brain automatically starts freaking out beyond the normal acceptable level of freaking out.

Bad things happen to people all the time...and when I say bad things, I mean little things like a flat tire, being late, spilling your coffee, car breaking down, or getting a speeding ticket.

But when my depression is bad – these things are enough to ruin my life for the next few weeks.

I obsess over them. I let them completely take over my day. I become hysterical and unreasonable.

Those who know me know I have terrible luck with cars...something is always wrong. Well, when my oil leaked out of my car this winter, I was irrationally upset.

My mind immediately goes to, "Well, this day is shot to hell". I let it ruin my entire day.

It's quite astonishing how one bad thing that is really no big deal can make such a huge impact on my mood. So, I try to get my logical brain to work and think rationally about the situation at hand. It's difficult but doable.

Instead of drowning myself in negativity – I try to focus on the positive things that happened that day. I got to spend more time with my husband even if it was out in the snow working on a car.

{Depression Confession #11}

Depression and anxiety manifest themselves physically for me.

As if feeling the emotions related to my depression and anxiety weren't bad enough, I also get the physical symptoms too.

I get migraines...a lot. I sleep too much. I eat everything in sight. I cry constantly. I get heart palpitations. Sometimes I can't poop while other times food goes right through me (another one of those awesome embarrassing facts about depression). My stomach will hurt, my arms and legs can go numb, and I sweat.

Anxiety feels like I can't breathe, and my heart is going 100 miles an hour while depression feels like my heart is going too slow to live. Often, I feel them both at the same time, if that's possible.

In high school people would complain because I "always" had a headache or a stomach ache...come to find out it was my depression and anxiety causing all of it. They eventually stopped asking me to do things with them because most of the time I couldn't anyway. But none of us knew what was really going on...that I was exhibiting signs of stress, depression and anxiety.

There are a lot of physical symptoms of depression and anxiety. If you are experiencing any of these – make an appointment with your primary care doctor to see if depression or anxiety is affecting your life.

{Depression Confession #12}

Chronic pain plays a huge factor in my depression.

In 2011, I was diagnosed with a bladder condition called interstitial cystitis (the lining of my bladder is deteriorating and has a feeling of a constant bladder infection) and pelvic floor dysfunction (the muscles in my pelvis are spasming constantly) both of which illicit pain. I also have chronic migraines.

Waking up in pain makes it even harder to fight my depression each morning. The pain interferes with daily life as does depression – so together they really ruin my day.

It's hard to get up and do my daily routine when my head is pounding, I can barely look at the clock to see the time. Or my pelvis hurts so bad that I can barely sit down at work.

With my depression I always feel like my brain hates me – well, with my chronic pain issues – I feel like my whole body hates me. It feels like I'm at war with my brain and body. Depression and chronic pain feed off of each other. When one is bad – the other usually flares. I get more migraines when I'm depressed, and I get depressed when I get the migraines. It's another vicious cycle that I'm lucky enough to get stuck in.

Having chronic pain can also lead to suicidal thoughts – just wanting the pain to be gone – not wanting to go through it anymore. That pain can be physical or emotional – sometimes both.

I learned a mindfulness technique that sometimes works for my pain – I used to clench and tighten my whole body fighting against the pain

– but with the help of a therapist, I was able to learn to "let it be". I learned to recognize that I was in pain, but that it would go away. When I stopped fighting it – the pain lessoned. I do the same thing with my anxiety. The technique doesn't always work, but it's made a huge difference in my life.

I do not let the chronic pain run my life. Just as I do not let my depression run my life.

{Depression Confession #13}

There is a difference between being sad and being depressed.

Sadness is being sad when something bad happens, after losing a job, a breakup, or losing a pet.

In my opinion, depression can be started by sadness, but it progresses past that into a feeling a hopelessness. Depression extends past the social normality of sadness. When sadness "lasts too long" it could be an indication of depression.

Sadness happens when something in life goes wrong. Depression is much more complicated. Like I said, it can start with something going wrong, but it goes further than that.

My depression is often present without a reason for being sad. I have also been sad and not depressed. The two are not interchangeable.

To treat sadness, sometimes all it takes is some chocolate ice cream and a funny movie...but depression is more complex. To treat it, a multi-faceted plan of attack is needed.

If you think your sadness could be beginning to change to a depression contact your primary care doctor for options.

{Depression Confession #14}

Depression is different for everyone

Everyone's journey with depression is different.

Some can get out of bed in the morning – others can't.

Some can keep a job – others can't.

Some take medications – others don't.

Some self-harm – others don't.

Some are suicidal – others aren't.

Some have more bad days than others.

Some have support systems – some don't.

Some go to talk therapy – others don't.

Some will reach out – others won't.

Some need hospitalization while others don't.

Some will stay in recovery and others will relapse.

Some turn to self-medicating – some don't.

Everyone's story is different and that's okay. Everyone's journey is different, unique and valid. My depression story is not the same as anyone else's. That's what makes it so difficult to understand and treat depression.

{Depression Confession #15}

Depression is NOT attention seeking.

This is a common misconception especially for young people who struggle with depression. It is common for people to say that they are just "doing this for attention".

Regardless of "why" they are displaying symptoms of depression – it should be taken seriously, and help should be sought.

When I was in high-school displaying symptoms of depression such as irritability, self-harm and unstable emotions, I was not doing it for attention. I was doing it because I didn't know how else to ask for help, and I didn't know how else to handle the emotions and feelings I was going through.

Even as an adult – I don't share my struggle with depression to get attention – I share it because I want others to know that they aren't alone. I share it because I want people to understand, and I want to educate people. And to be honest...sharing my story – getting it out there and off my chest helps me to understand it myself. Instead of hiding it – I don't have to pretend as much. I can be real.

No matter what the "reason" for someone's depression, it's important they get the help they need from a doctor or mental health professional. Dismissing the signs and disregarding the symptoms could lead to a mental health crisis. The assumption that someone is displaying these characteristics for attention can be damaging.

{Depression Confession #16}

My depression keeps me from living my actual life.

What I mean by this is that I spend so much time worrying, fretting and stressing over what could be or might happen, that, I forget to live in the moment. Honestly...I forget how to live.

I forget that I'm living and breathing here...today...right now.

How does one forget that they are alive? I really don't know...but I do. I feel like I'm walking through my life just to get to the end of each day, to say that I made it another day.

I've recently been working on being with myself and showing up for me...for my life. Instead of going through the motions and just "making it" each day.

I choose to be present in my life for myself and for those around me.

How does one do this?

I breathe. I breathe deep and long to remind myself that I am alive. I take breaks from the noisy social media and television life that our society has come to love. I drink my tea and take walks to strengthen my body and mind. I focus on self-care and self-love to help keep my brain healthy.

Instead of sleeping the day away, I wake up and start the day right...by being with myself and my dogs for a few minutes before turning to my phone to see what I've missed in the last 8 hours I was asleep. I just try my best to be my best.

{Depression Confession #17}

My depression makes me a very good actress.

I've spent a lot of my life fighting depression and trying to hide it from others. I didn't want to "bring others down". Honestly, it was easier to hide it then to explain my depression and sadness to others.

So, my smile was large, and my laughter was heard. I pretended to be present in conversations. I was always the first to show concern for those around me and was always willing to help in any way I can.

What people didn't realize is the screaming in my head, the tears before bed, and the pain searing every inch of my body. I let them see what they "needed" to see – the smiles, the laughter, the put together face of makeup and happiness.

When I was asked, "How are you?", I would always answer, "Good!", when inside I wanted to answer, "Terrible!".

It was exhausting to be "someone else", but that's what I did – I pretended to be someone I wasn't.

I'm not sure what changed – but one day I decided I wasn't going to hide it anymore.

Once I shared my journey with depression with those around me, I was able to stop pretending. I was able to honestly answer the question, "How are you?" Now I answer it truthfully. "I'm struggling today" or "I'm having a good day today!" or "I'm not sure yet how I feel today."

I don't have to act anymore, and it feels like a weight off my chest and a freedom I can't even explain.

Just like I said in the previous confession – I don't share my story for attention – I share it because it helps me control my depression and help others.

{Depression Confession #18}

I don't have to be strong all the time.

This is one I struggle with the most because I have always felt like I needed to be strong. Strong for my mom and my sister after losing my dad. Strong for my patients who are sick and in pain. Strong for my friends and strangers who come to me with losses or struggles of their own.

I have been strong for so long. One of my favorite quotes is:

"Stay Strong. Stay Brave. Stay True. Stay You."

I created this quote during my second partial hospitalization program. But after time, I realized that I don't have to stay strong...I don't even have to stay brave. But I do have stay true and I have to stay me. I must STAY.

It's okay to not be okay –it's okay to cry – to let my guard down sometimes. It's okay to break down occasionally. All these feelings are valid and important.

So, while I will continue to remind myself to "Stay Strong", I will always know that it's okay to feel things. It's important to feel things and not hide them away in order to be strong.

{Depression Confession #19}

Depression is not me. I am not depression.

I have depression. Depression does not have me.

Depression feels like it can take over my entire life, my mind and body. It can make me feel like depression is my personality – that I am depression.

But I am NOT.

I have an illness. I have depression. It affects many aspects of my life and some days it may be the only focus, but I am so much more than my depression.

I am kind. I am honest. I am beautiful. I help people. I laugh. I am a wife. I am a daughter. I am a sister. I am an ultrasound tech. I am a mental health advocate. I am more than depression.

&& so are you!

Depression Confession Extras:

"Even if it looks on the outside that I'm ok, I'm not. I may have my hair done and makeup on. I may put a smile on my face and attempt to act completely normal. The part people don't see is what's in my head and in my heart. That I'm dying inside and struggling to hold it all together. That just because it seems like a good day, doesn't mean it is. My depression is constantly in my head and heart. My anxiety is non-stop and I'm always on edge waiting for the next bad thing to happen. Judging me by the outside isn't okay because inside I'm dying. All the time." – Bridgette B.

"Getting out of bed is all I have energy for some days. When telling someone I have depression I do not say it for sympathy; I say it for the possibility of understanding. Depression is not easy – some days I want loved ones near to comfort me and other days I can't stand being loved by others because I don't feel I deserve it/them. I feel guilty sharing when I'm depressed with loved ones as I think it brings all those around me down too." – Alyssa B.

"I feel guilty for experiencing depression and for having thoughts about hating my life because I know that I have a life that others would dream of." – Sarah B.

"My Dearest Depression,

Are you my foe? My friend? What I am certain of is you are my constant, steadfast life companion. I have a lifetime of memories with you. In moments of joy, you warn me of the fickle, fleeting nature of such an emotion. Joy is unlike you - she does not linger, stalk or haunt me as you do. No one is quite like you, my loyal companion.

In my moments of deepest despair or sorrow, you remind me how much deeper you can push me. Ever the overachiever, right? In my moments of greatest achievement, you unfailingly warn me of the impending exposure as a fraud and the fatal nature of the fall from such heights. What would I do without your loving reminders?

Every second of every day, you never cease to whisper your warnings. You are there when I wake, when I eat, when I work, when I make love and when I sleep - if you deign it proper for me to sleep. To be fair, sometimes in your infinite benevolence, you bless me with sleep. Sleep so heavy and deep that I forgo food, hygiene, work and family. Sleep so sweet I start imagining & wishing for eternal sleep.

Will we be together forever? Why do I both dread and love the thought of losing you? You flit through my mind at will like memories of a great lost love. Am I Heathcliff and you are my Catherine? Am I willing you to haunt me forever? Without my constant companion, who am I? Without my constant companion, who can I be?

Your faithful servant,
S"

"Depression, a word I heard often. A word you hear so often that when it hits after your mom passes and the dust settles, you cannot call it by its name. You start to realize what it is when it hits after dropping kids off at school you crawl back into bed and getting up is hard to do. When you see your kids clean a room in minutes while it takes you all week to do. Sure, some days are good. There is clarity. Then the other days, the brain fog comes in. You know you have an event and it takes you all day to get ready for it. That's if you even make it out the door. Depression was never part of my life other than my father having it. That is until I lost my mother. Now I know what it is called by name. However long or short it chooses to stay...Depression sucks." – Melissa Z.

"I have said many times that things have changed for the better. However, lately, when I look in the mirror, I have a strange feeling like it isn't even me. The job I used to call my "heart and soul" is now something I can't bear. I'm not sure if I want to pursue being a nurse anymore – a lifelong dream of mine. My divorce will be final in exactly one month – this girl who used to strive for true love no longer believes she is worthy, recounting all the times she tried so hard to love the wrong man. I tell myself ugly lies about how stupid, useless and lost I am, because "I'm going to die anyway". I could go on but the gist of it is just how badly I've lost who I am. I once was a driven lively and happy gal. Now I am despondent, sad, scared and irritable." – Miranda V.

"I miss my friends terribly but when they call and invite me to do things, I can't bear the thought of leaving the house. I look at my art supplies and long to paint but can't pick up a brush. I haven't played my piano in 7 years. I gave up on my dream of a classroom of my own because I look at other teachers and think I can't possibly do all they do. Even though... yes... I can... but the voices in my head are so loud they drown the truth. Sometimes I seem like the life of the party at work, but inside...I am SCREAMING...and want to get in my car and leave everyone and everything...as I am sick of being blamed for something I don't know how to change. I am sick of people getting mad at me and accusing me of not appreciating my life, but they do not understand I don't think I deserve to be happy." – Cynthia H.

"What I show and how I pretend to be is totally different on the inside. What they see is not what I am on the inside. Depression keeps me cold and in a dark place. I feel like being alone is safer because I don't have to pretend, I'm okay and fake it. But when I wake up and I just feel like I'm carrying more than I can, but I just push to handle it. The anxiety creeps up when my depression is full force and it makes it seem like it's even hard to breathe. I just can't wait till I'm back in my safe place and away from everyone because they just don't understand, or it makes me feel as if I'm weak. Feeling as if you're broken and fragile but try and never feel complete. Your safe place becomes a place where you're alone, and you feel that there's no judgement, and you can be real with yourself looking in the mirror and realizing your emotions are out of control when you're broken, but you can't do that in real life because people see you as weak. Hiding behind a mask hides what or who you really feel like on the inside. Hide the scars, tears, and pain so you look normal on the outside, but you're scarred, broken, and fragile. For me personally, I don't know when or how it's going to hit me but when it does, it takes me to a place that I have to fight to crawl out of. I often find myself walking into the light when I turn, I see that dark comfortable tunnel it's a safe place to be sometimes, even though it doesn't make sense. Being labeled weak adds to my own struggles and makes my insecurities rise and makes me question myself. It's an awful place to be. So, when I'm not so fragile, I feel better, strong and like I can take on anything. When I'm weak, I just can't." – Annette B.

"I only appear to have it all together. Most days getting out of bed is a major victory. Even on medication, the urge to cry is strong. Saying I'm fine is a lie...I'm not. I don't want to feel this way. I miss me.... or the me I think I used to be." – Tracy H.

"Depression keeps me from being present for my kids. When I think about it, I feel sick and guilty, which just makes me more depressed. It's a horrible cycle." – Brienne R.

"I'd rather stay in my room, in bed, sleeping. When I get up, I don't want to do anything. I feel like showering or other normal activities takes too much energy or I just don't care. I also, distance myself from my family including my kids. I can get into such a deep hole it feels like I'll never get out. Most days I only leave my room if I have to go to work." – Josette S.

"When it gets bad, it combines with my OCD to distract me from doing work or any of the things I need to do to better myself. What I'm depressed about becomes the focus of my brain like a broken record; while I do far better now with the tools I have, it still can ruin an otherwise good day for me due to one event." – John F.

"Mine is just when I have a lot on my plate and no one to share it with but is usually in full force when my daughter is suffering." – Karen C.

"Somedays it's hard to physically leave my apartment or go out with friends even though we made plans. I don't like the pressure of faking like I'm okay or having fun when all I want to do is lay in my bed. The darkest days make happiness feel so very far away...worlds away. On the days I feel like I'm drowning in my depression I wonder if it will ever get better or be like this forever. I worry others don't want to be around me or view me as weak because of my mental illness. Somedays are really draining. Being around people and trying to function sucks the life out of me." – Derrica D.

"I'll pretend to be asleep or "accidentally" sleep in so that I don't have to handle something" – Meg R.

"My depression has actually caused my work performance at work to plummet. I just couldn't get it together. I thought there was no point because no one would miss me if I left. I still struggle with it off and on, but my husband has been my rock and it isn't as much of a struggle now." – Molly C.

"Sometimes I have to nap, or more like lay stiff on the couch for hours, to keep myself safe, alive, to keep from hurting myself. It's different than when I'm paralyzed by my anxiety, it's when I can't shake the horrible thoughts, it's hard to explain, I just know I have to go lay down to be safe and stay;" – Amber G.

"My grandma was diagnosed with dementia. She sits deep in her mind and lives in a world she paints, despite what's happening around her. I naively try to bring her things to jog her memory and bring her back to me. More times than not, I sob in my car knowing I can't break those walls and will only be living around her world, not in it. It's much like my depression. I sit deep in my mind, my walls are painted grey, and I try, naively, to pull myself out only to fail. Not because I can't break the gray, bleak walls – but because I am trapped within them. My depression is isolation, it's anxiety, it's not having the fight to show up for your own life." – Lacee S.

"Depression for me is pretending to be someone that I am not in the moment. I'm that person who you always see with a smile. Who laughs at every little thing...who says good morning/afternoon without hesitation. Who asks how you are? But on the inside, I'm screaming, I'm crying. When no one is near, I'm in a zombie state of mind. Depression is fighting every day to brush my hair or teeth, to stay focused when driving. Just once I would like to truthful to the people around me when someone asks how I'm doing. I always say, "I'm fine." And keep walking because I cannot look them in the eye. I feel like I'm scratching myself from the inside to get out of the shell of a body. I cannot explain it any other way. I feel some days like I'm dying inside, that the darkness is consuming my mind, body and spirit. Meds don't help, they just make me feel worse, so I just try to stay busy, so I can keep my mind focused and I try to help other people because that makes me the happiest when other people smile because of something I've said or done." – Jessica D.

"I have been dealing with depression and anxiety for almost a year now, and boy has it been a ride. The biggest struggle that I deal with on a daily basis is comparison. More specifically, comparing my mental health to others battling the same fight. I compare others who have been hospitalized and have been to the brink of suicide to myself who, in my eyes, doesn't have it as bad. I have never been hospitalized, I have never attempted suicide, I struggle day by day not hour by hour. Most times I just feel like I need to suck it up and be grateful for what I have because others have it worse than I do. But in reality, it's all the same. We all struggle, we all know what it's like, we all just take it at a different pace. That is what I'm learning. It's a hard lesson to swallow, but I'm learning. And I want anyone else who thinks the same way I do to know that no matter how silly you feel about what you are feeling is absolutely and completely okay. We are all warriors and we all will fight our fight and we will be victorious. Keep fighting." – Tabby P.

"Depression is rolling over in bed and seeing the clock flash 11:36 but you can't get your body to get yourself out of bed. Being born in a family that demands perfection then realizing you're the overweight one who never has any money. Depression is seeing your grandparents dote on their perfect granddaughter and it's not you. In fact, often times hearing them talk about her like she is their only grandchild. You want to leave the house and hang out with your friends, but instead make an excuse to why you can't at the last minute-then slowly watching them call less and slip away. It's the inner struggle with yourself to live your life and be happy and fun but again it's 11:36 and I can't get out of bed" – Katlyn T.

"Being on the other side: Early on in my career as a hospital worker, I was part of the trauma team. I literally saw hundreds of traumas, but nothing affected me as much as suicide attempts. See, I've fought my own demons from time to time and often thought I had ruined my own life at different points. The lowest point was when going through my divorce and feeling fairly hopeless...Two days post-divorce, a trauma call comes in. I race to the ER trauma room with O Negative blood and gathered some details. Nothing could have prepared me for what came through the door. His suicide attempt was gruesome and violent. This young guy had broken up with his girlfriend and obviously could not bear the pain anymore. He died the next day from his injuries. I have had many dark days since this day, but I always remember this young man. I remember the smells of this day and the screams of his family. Life is tough, but it is so worth staying around for. "– Mark E.

"Into the Darkness
Into the darkness my soul
does soar
Like the wings of the
dragonfly.
Never resting to catch my
Breath
Longing for the days
gone by.

No one hears the
dragonfly
As it flutters to and fro
For the ones that are next
to you
Are always on the go.
As my soul makes its
journey
In the race that we call life
I no longer can be silent
Or my soul in be in strife.

For my family to see me
struggle
Is really not that fair,
But to see me leave this
life
Would be too much to
bear.

So, I will tell my story
To those close to me
For I suffer from
depression

And I am not the only one
you see.

This world turns its blind
eye
To this disease that takes
so many
For the subject is taboo
And joked about plenty.

As my life span is half
over
I look back and see
The child that is inside of
me
Is the place I would rather
be.

A time of no worries
No pain or guilt be found
But those times are now
behind me
And never to be unbound.

As my story continues on
And my voice becomes a
roar
My soul that is on the
dragonfly
Will into the darkness
soar."
-    Shawn T.

"I feel like I'm always failing everyone. Failing as a wife, mother, daughter, sister, etc. How can you get compliments from everyone and still pick apart everything you do and everything you don't. I yell at my kids when I get irritable or stressed and then I ponder how I'm damaging them. I've seen it myself. Everyone gets stressed and yells but I just feel like to me what's failure as a mom that I should be their safe place and I push everyone away. That's probably why I don't have any friends. Even in my happiest those tricky little monsters (thoughts) sneak in here or there – worry that my husband will leave or cheat or secretly hate and resent me for things, paranoia that this is too good to be true or that something bad will happen. Do I just try to keep pushing them out and keep focusing on the happy things in life? Because worrying about those things will only steal today's joy. I've tried several different counselors over the years and haven't found one that helped. I rely a lot on my faith during difficult times. I pray and read scripture." – Miranda D.

"I live chronically ill, every time I "flare" from Crohn's, I slip into the biggest depression that drags me into the deepest darkest hole. It's like clockwork, I spiral out of control in my health and soon after I lose it mentally. Talking helps, friends forcing themselves into my life or home helps. Just being there for me, being lazy and watching Netflix together, they're there for me, and that's what we need when we slip in that hole. Depression when you have flare after flare, surgery and more flare, or complications that arise, it feels like the struggle will never end and at times it can be completely and utterly exhausting, physically and mentally. You end up getting lack of sleep and that just adds to the crazy mess of depression. You never know what anyone goes through, so if you have a friend admitting they struggle with depression, DO NOT IGNORE that conversation. Be there and be aware when they start making excuses not to come out, and force yourself back into their life when they try and push you out, trust me...it helps." – Shannon C.

"When asked as an icebreaker "tell us one of your hobbies," it is always so difficult to think of even one. When someone asked "tell me a depression confession," now that is something I can come up with without any thought. Out of the thousands I have, what do I choose?

The most heartbreaking one yet. Postpartum depression. I have always had depression, but what that meant for me was that I often didn't know how to make myself happy but spent way too much time trying to make others happy.

Then came my son. When they laid him on my chest, I didn't want to hold him, when they tried to have me breastfeed, I didn't want to, when I tried to wake up in the night and take care of him I couldn't. The amount of times you are reminded you how much you "should" love your newborn child are endless. The doctor acts shocked when you don't breastfeed, your in-laws are confused when you would rather cry alone in your room than be in a room full of people oohing and awwwing at your baby.

The truth is I didn't love him and at 5 months old somedays I wonder if I even do now. Do we have a space to say these things out loud? Not that I have found. My husband listens, but I don't dare tell anyone else that I often wish I didn't have a child. I watched my mother and friends struggle to conceive and here I am wishing I hadn't?

Depression, you are the horrible friend I can't seem to stand up to. Someday I will, but for now I will hold on to the hope that one morning I will wake up and you will be gone." – Anonymous

"I tell myself for months that I am fine, because I'm not overwhelmed with sadness. I don't even feel that sad at all. I'm just tired. But it goes down from there. I start eating less because I'm so exhausted all the time that making food seems like too much work. Then I eat even less, because even getting food that's already made is a chore. I have less and less motivation, until all I care about is finding more time to sleep because I. Am. So. Exhausted. All. The. Time. So, I stop showering at night and tell myself I'll shower in the morning. Except, I don't. And then I can barely make myself shower once a week and I'm embarrassed that I'm so tired and lazy that I can't even bathe. But I'm fine, because I'm not sad or suicidal. I'm just tired. But actually, I'm fine because I don't feel anything. Just perpetual exhaustion, and a general sense of irritability. Everything makes me vaguely annoyed, and it makes me snap sometimes. But I don't want to focus on how tired I am, and feel nothing instead. And it takes me so long to realize what's happening, and then even more time to finally make myself do something. It's taking baby steps like making sure I always have snacks to eat at work, like string cheese and goldfish because they are the easiest thing for me to eat. Then making myself take the time to take a bath because it's relaxing and I know I'll take an actual shower afterwards. It's spending a bunch of money on a fitness class because then I feel inclined to go, and it'll at least get me out and doing something physical once a week. And it literally becomes a "fake it till you make it" scenario, and I have to force myself to take these baby steps before I can finally feel some sense of normalcy again. It is a literal battle with myself with the "sick" part of myself fighting to stay stagnant, while the logical part of myself furiously screams that I am more than this. I can beat this." – Monica A

Anxiety Admissions

{Anxiety Admission #1}

Anxiety presents itself in many ways.

When my anxiety flares, I literally feel so much that I cannot even tell you what I am feeling. So, when people ask me, "What is wrong?" I don't have an answer because I have no idea other than "It's my anxiety."

I have difficulty managing my emotions – crying when I don't want to, for example.

I get antsy/agitated – I cannot sit still but don't know where to go or what to do with myself.

I get irritable – I get angry over the smallest, insignificant things. I know it's irrational, but it doesn't stop my brain.

I get frustrated because I have no idea why my brain is doing this.

I chew my nails to the quick without even knowing I'm doing it.

I feel fear/panic because my brain is telling me this isn't going to end. Even though I know it will, my brain is incapable of rational thinking.

I can't get to sleep easily. My mind races a million miles a minute with everything I should have gotten done that day and all that I have to do the next day.

I have difficulty paying attention and focusing. I am "all over the place".

I over plan, stress and worry over situations and have very high expectations for myself that are sometimes not realistic. I have a high desire to be in control of everything around me (which is also not realistic).

Anxiety is my brain racing through every single possible thought that I have in the blink of an eye. If I thought depression is exhausting – anxiety is even worse.

{Anxiety Admission #2}

Panic Attacks are straight from hell.

They typically only last a few minutes but feel like they last a lifetime. Time seems to slow down, but my heart is racing. My brain races through every possible thought. I usually start to hyperventilate and get chest pains. I cry and shake. To say panic attacks are straight from hell is an understatement in my eyes. They are so much worse.

I can sometimes talk myself out of them if I catch it early enough – reminding myself that I'm alive and I'm okay (after practice and many failed attempts). Other times I need assistance. I have my anti-anxiety medication, but I try to use other methods first. I have a couple different apps on my phone that guide me in meditation/breathing exercises. I also try different grounding techniques such as naming 5 things I can touch around me, 5 things I can smell or taste or hear. It seems silly at first – but it really does help!

I also try to remain there with the anxiety. I know it sounds backwards. What I mean is – I don't fight it. I let it come and let it be...I know that it is only a feeling and that it will pass. I recognize that I'm having symptoms of a panic attack or a bad anxiety day and I am able to allow those feelings to be with me, without them overwhelming me. This is the same method that I use to handle my chronic pain. It is not an easy thing to learn and definitely not an easy thing to do.

{Anxiety Admission #3}

Anxiety has many triggers but sometimes there isn't one.

I have generalized anxiety which means that a lot of the time my anxiety doesn't have a specific trigger. My anxiety often starts when I get overwhelmed at home or at work.

It makes me so frustrated/mad when I cannot pinpoint what I am anxious about – all I know is that I can't sit still, I can't breathe right, and I have no idea why. My husband and others will frequently ask what it is that I'm anxious about – but I have nothing to tell them. I just say that "I don't know". This then makes it difficult for them to help me. They don't know if they should leave me alone or give me a hug, if they should keep quiet or say something. If only they realized that I have no idea what I am anxious about. It makes me even more anxious that I don't know what I'm anxious about!

I do have some triggers that make my anxiety worse that I've been able to identify – large social gatherings, driving to places I don't know, and being late are my top three. But most often my anxiety will manifest itself during a typical day with no obvious triggers at all.

{Anxiety Admission #4}

Depression and Anxiety often occur together.

If you're lucky like me, you have both depression and anxiety affecting your life.

Depression which can makes me feel nothing and anxiety which makes me feel everything – they tend to wreak havoc on my life.

It's a vicious cycle of feeling nothing and being depressed to then feeling overly anxious and back again.

One day I can be so depressed that I don't get off the couch, and the next day, I am extremely anxious because I wasted the whole previous day doing nothing. Then I get depressed because I didn't do anything and anxious because I'm depressed.

I struggle with the ups and downs of having both depression and anxiety, but I get through it by relying on my support system to keep me together. I also work on identifying my symptoms to help me keep track of triggers and patterns. I can then work on those triggers and patterns with my therapist.

{Anxiety Admission #5}

Anxiety tricks your brain to think something bad will happen.

Anxiety has an awesome habit of sneaking into every part of my life just like the depression does. When things seem to be going well and I'm happy, anxiety will then show itself and make me think that I'm doing something wrong or that something bad is going to happen. Then starts the awful anxiety of non-stop racing thoughts and panic.

Anxiety isn't fair – it comes when you least expect it and takes over your mind.

Anxiety makes me believe that I am not good enough, that I am doing something wrong or that something terrible will happen. Anxiety has its way of being the sole focus of my brain – it's a tunnel vision where everything is exaggerated and unrealistic.

This is another instance of my brain having two parts to it – the logical part and the chaos part. The chaos part just takes over and runs amok. It takes time for my logical brain to get back in the driver's seat.

{Anxiety Admission #6}

Anxiety makes me irritable – to the point where it impacts my relationships.

When my anxiety is unusually high, my irritability also gets very high. I turn into the nagging, yelling, wife and treat my husband poorly. I will get upset over the smallest, insignificant things.

For example, after a hard day at work and I came home to the house being even the slightest bit messy I would become extremely angry – when in reality – there is nothing to be angry about. We are humans and we live in a house – it can't be perfect 100% of the time. I would get irrationally upset if we were running late for something because being late and driving are two of my anxiety triggers.

It took us a long time to recognize that my irritability was related to my anxiety. Now that we know, I am able to work on my anxiety and it reduces the irritability as well.

Anxiety Admission Extras:

"Living with depression is bad enough, but when you add high functioning anxiety into the mix, it's a whole new beast. There are days I feel everything and nothing all at once, days that I feel so empty even though I know I have a lot going for me. I love my life and all of the people in it, but sometimes my depression convinces me that I am not enough, or that I can't do things. There are days that my depression makes me feel like there is no point, days that even the smallest tasks seem impossible. During depressive episodes, even things like taking a shower or remembering to brush my hair is overwhelming. If there is one thing that I have been able to hold onto during the darkest of times is that THIS TOO SHALL PASS! Though it may feel like it's never going to end, I know that stars cannot shine without darkness!" – Liz B.

"I've lost almost 70lbs this year because my anxiety makes me so nauseated, I can hardly keep anything down. I even ended up in the hospital for malnutrition. Everyone tells me how good I look now." – Meg R.

"I suffer from anxiety/panic attacks. I was in ER three times in a year because I thought I was having a heart attack. I now take Xanax as needed and a daily depression/anxiety medication. Every time I went to the ER because I was having chest pains or couldn't breathe. I felt crazy! Like people thought I was faking! Now thankfully I know what the chest tightening and heavy chest is and I take a very small dose of Xanax until it passes. The crazy thing to me is it will happen when I don't feel panicked at all no explanation" – Tressa S.

"I'm a therapist. I know how to ward off depression and anxiety, right? I teach other people how to manage their symptoms, so I must be symptom-free, right? Not so much. I've struggled with depression and anxiety since I was a teen. I once thought about crashing my car into a telephone pole, but never acted on the thought. 16 years have passed since my teenage brain had that thought. I've been in therapy for myself for almost all of those 16 years. I've been with my current therapist for 9 years. In my mid-20's I was put on medication and with some trial and error finally found the magic combination for me and have been relatively stable for several years. On June 10, 2016, my grandmother died. It was expected. I actually flew home to say goodbye to her before Christmas 2015. Even though it was expected, the news hit me hard. I left work crying immediately after my mother called me with the news. My job was pretty awful and I just couldn't go back. I was burnt out and depressed. My psychiatrist put me out on FMLA leave for 4 weeks and then I quit. During that first month, I was a mess. I couldn't even decide for myself to brush my teeth, change my clothes or do anything but lay on the couch and watch daytime TV and Golden Girls reruns late into the night. My husband had to literally flip a coin to make those basic decisions for me. I eventually found a part time job at a college bookstore, and that, combined with networking with other therapists, brought me back to life. I was hired as a therapist again in November 2016.

I'm happy to report that I have not experienced another major depressive episode since, but my anxiety still rears its ugly head at times. I call it "My Anxiety Monster" and I've even drawn his picture, per my therapist's guidance. He looks kind of like an angry, purple SpongeBob. He eats and grows by telling me how much I have to do and how little time I have to do it and/or how incapable or unprepared I am to do the things on my list. I have not yet "made friends" with My Anxiety Monster. I look for evidence that counters his negative comments about me and then I pick something small to start my list. If I need to clean the kitchen, I start by loading the dishwasher and then the items that need to go from the countertop to their home upstairs get put at the bottom of the stairs, to take up on my next trip. Since, I started using guided meditations on a daily basis, my Anxiety Monster is not as strong as he used to be. Some days are harder than others, but I am a fighter. I didn't give up when I was 16 and I'm not giving up now. I am aware of my anxiety and I cope with it. I use motivational quotes like vitamins to keep me alive. I can't choose a single favorite, there are so many, but for now I leave you with this: Be brave and keep going. "– Anonymous

"For me I can't even count how many times I ended up to the emergency room because I didn't know what was happening. I thought my heart was stopping or the numerous times I just collapsed. Waking to the paramedics over me. Not understanding what was the cause, I remember thinking I was going to die but for the longest time I wanted to die after I lost my daughter Brittanie but when I was rushed into the hospital not knowing what was happening it startled me. I realized I wanted to live, so I worked hard to learn how to breathe and cope thru the anxiety." – Annette B.

"My anxiety tells me no one likes me and they're just being nice because they're nice people not because they like me. My depression and anxiety convinces me frequently I'm toxic to be around, so I succumb to it and secluded myself." – Heather M

Suicidal Thoughts

{Depression Confession #20}

Suicidal thoughts happen with my depression.

I often feel so much pain that it seems the only way out of the pain is to end my life. It's a tunnel vision of pain and relentless thoughts of hopelessness, loneliness and sadness. It's a constant barrage of self-hatred and loathing. The pain is so extreme that I can't even see straight, let alone think coherently. I only think about dying. That I don't want to be on this earth anymore – that I'm not worth it. I've struggled with these thoughts at various points in my journey with depression – most often when my meds were not regulated or when I drink too much.

When these thoughts invade my brain, I used to hide them and pretend they weren't there. I didn't want to believe that I was thinking them – even though it was obvious. When I hid them, they would fester and force themselves that much more into my brain.

I used to hide them but now I reach out…I make an extra therapy appointment; I call my psychiatrist, or go to the emergency room if needed. I also keep my house safe. I have a safety plan. I avoid spending time alone if I'm having suicidal thoughts – I surround myself with friends and family (even when I would rather be alone) to help keep me safe until I can get stabilized.

If you fight suicidal thoughts like I do – be sure to talk to your doctor, therapist or psychiatrist. If you have suicidal thoughts right now, call the National Prevention Lifeline at 1-800-273-8255 or text "TALK" to 741-741. If you are in immediate crisis, call 911 or go to the nearest emergency department.

{Depression Confession #21}

Not all people who have depression have suicidal thoughts.

Many people who live with depression never experience suicidal thoughts or ideation. This is a GREAT thing! I wouldn't wish those thoughts on my worst enemy.

Just because you have depression does not mean you are suicidal.

This is something that society really needs to learn – there is a stigma associated with saying you have depression and people then think you are a fragile person that may kill yourself if they say the wrong thing.

In fact, most of the time I am not suicidal with my depression. My depression is often solo – no suicidal thinking at all. Like I said, my suicidal thoughts *usually* come if I miss a dose of medication or become too intoxicated.

{Depression Confession #22}

Suicidal thoughts can invade my mind when I least expect it.

In the previous confession I stated that I usually have suicidal thoughts after missing a dose of medication or become too intoxicated, however, if my depression is left unchecked, meaning I am not on my medication, suicidal thoughts tend to become more common for me.

Suicidal thoughts do not just happen when I'm alone at home at night. They can show up when I'm spending time with my friends or family. They happen when I'm driving. They even happen during the day at work!

I've had to leave work once because the suicidal thoughts were so strong, I needed immediate intervention. I was able to contact my boss and co-workers to help keep me safe while other arrangements were made.

It's hard to tell people that I'm suicidal at times when others are having a great time or a normal day. But it's important to recognize the thoughts and address them no matter where I am.

If you are having these thoughts – be sure to talk to your doctor, therapist or psychiatrist. If you have suicidal thoughts right now, call the National Prevention Lifeline at 1-800-273-8255 or text "TALK" to 741-741. If you are in immediate crisis, call 911 or go to the nearest emergency department.

{Depression Confession #23}

Self-Harm is not always an indication of suicidal thoughts.

In high school, I was a cutter – not because I wanted to die but because it was something that I could control. I controlled the pain instead of the pain controlling me.

As an adult, I would scratch my arms or thighs. I was never suicidal when I self-harmed. It was just a coping mechanism for me... although it is not the healthiest coping mechanism, which is why I started therapy and exercising – to find a better way to cope with the emotions I was facing.

When I was hospitalized, I was taught to color mandalas. That coloring can bring your brain from a state of chaos back to a state of focus and calm. It is a wonderful coping mechanism that truly helps me when I am overwhelmed. It is so helpful to me that I got a mandala tattooed on my thigh so that I would always have something to color instead of hurting myself.

Although self-harm is not always an indication of suicidal thoughts – it should not be dismissed easily. It IS an indication that something is wrong. Whether it's the inability to cope with pain or a true act of suicidal thinking it should be taken seriously.

{Depression Confession #24}

Suicidal thoughts aren't always specifically about killing oneself.

Most of the time I am not thinking "I want to kill myself". I am not always thinking about ways to die. I mostly just think – I don't want to be here. My thoughts are commonly -

> I want to sleep forever.

> I just don't want to wake up.

> I wish it was all over.

> I wish the pain would just end.

> I wish I was never born.

> The world wouldn't miss me anyway.

These count as suicidal thoughts. All these thoughts resonate to the same thing… "I don't want to be here anymore."

If you are having these thoughts – be sure to talk to your doctor, therapist or psychiatrist. If you have suicidal thoughts right now, call the National Prevention Lifeline at 1-800-273-8255 or text "TALK" to 741-741. If you are in immediate crisis, call 911 or go to the nearest emergency department.

{Depression Confession #25}

Keeping my house safe is vital to keeping me alive.

Even when I am not having suicidal thoughts, we keep our house safe.

We have all firearms in a safe that I don't have the combination to. My anxiety medications with the potential for overdose are also in the safe to be given as needed by my husband.

I developed a safety plan multiple times throughout my hospitalizations and recovery. It helps to keep it visible and I make sure that my husband and family are familiar with it too. It's a small step towards keeping myself safe when suicidal thoughts come.

See my sample safety plan:

Warning Signs: Irritability, crying, hyperventilating, panic attacks, drinking more, self-harming (scratching/cutting), thoughts of dying or killing myself.

Coping Strategies: Grounding (name every object in front of you), hold an ice cube in hand, 4x4 breathing (breathe in for 4 secs, hold for 4 secs, let it out for 4 secs, breathe in for 4 secs), coloring

People to Call for Help: My mom or sister, my husband, my therapist, my friends. Or go to the nearest emergency department if in immediate crisis.

{Depression Confession #26}

My suicidal thoughts are most often ambiguous - meaning part of me wants to live and part of me wants to die.

I've had multiple episodes of suicidal thoughts on my journey with depression.

Every time, I did not want to die...I just wanted the pain to end. It's a battle in my brain trying to find another way out. It's important to focus and pursue the part of me that wants to live and create distance from the part that wants to die.

How do I do that?

I do things that make me happy and make me feel alive. I go for walks and take in the sunshine...or the rain...or the snow and remember that I am breathing and living for a reason. I see my therapist to talk through my thought processes and to change my distorted thinking to more helpful thinking.

I stay away from sitting at home alone and drinking because I know those two things will reinforce the distorted thinking.

Focusing on the parts of me that want to live helps make the part of me that wants to die get smaller and smaller.

Depression Confession Extras:

"My husband, Josh, has suffered from depression and suicidal thoughts since he was 7. He had a teacher tell him he was worthless and stupid one afternoon at school. His mom found him after he attempted suicide that night and he was admitted to in-patient treatment three different times for a total of 3-4 months. He is 34 now and while he still struggles with suicidal thoughts and depression, he looks at our daughter and he finds himself saying, "This little girl right here is the reason I am still here." – Molly & Josh C.

"My experience with depression has been a constant battle, since the day I was diagnosed at 12 years old. I've battled against multiple people who don't believe my feelings are real, and ask why I can't just get over it. I've battled with friends and family who feel that my medication is a cop-out; that I'm not facing my problems. I've battled with myself every time I see a bottle of pills or wash a kitchen knife or drive on a winding road. A battle to keep myself alive. My fight may not be orthodox, but it's what works for me. I subject myself to hours of pain under ink, needles, and metal to try to make beautiful the body that I so often hate. To feel something, anything, even if it's excruciating pain. I create playlists of songs screaming the emotions I cannot describe myself. I think about what song would be played for me if I were to die. I also realize that I have a purpose here, and that there are people depending on me. On my toughest days, I think of my nephew, who wouldn't understand why Auntie is suddenly gone. Most days, what is keeping me around is other people, and not myself. Most often, I would love to be gone. Maybe someday, I'll be able to stay for myself. Until then, I still have something keeping me here." – Tessa N.

"As a teacher you see me as a happy, positive, role-model for your children. What you don't see are my mania symptoms at the end of the day that make me sleep 13 hours a night, or the days where I can't sleep because my brain wants to do laundry or check my bank account at 3AM. You don't see when I think about killing myself at lunch, because I have the time. But I stay, I try, I fight, because I love your children, I love my nephews, my siblings. I stay because my family have gone through this before.
Sincerely,
A fighting teacher"

"I have always struggled with depression throughout my life. After my fiancé passed away, I remember driving to someone's house. I was at a red light and a semi-truck was driving through the green light, and I remember thinking if I pull out in front of this truck there is a pretty good chance I'll die and then get to be with him forever. It was the oddest feeling because I wasn't feeling suicidal, more just considering the idea of not being existent anymore. I thought about death all the time, and how not having to be existent would be so beautiful because I would be happy forever with him." – Alyssa B.

"I got to the point that I felt worthless, I didn't like myself, I only saw my flaws. I was negative to myself and to others. I thought of and went through the steps of being destructive. I had terrible mood swings and felt unloved and unimportant by everyone. I completely understand why people die by suicide. My brother left us on Jan 1st, 2015, that way. I had no idea he suffered from depression, (well, not to his severity anyway)." – Cheryl R.

"I was suicidal. I couldn't think of anything else other than dying. I didn't want to be on this planet anymore. I literally thought about dying every day. It was a dark and hopeless time. I was hospitalized until these thoughts went away with therapy and medication." – Anonymous

Stigma

{Depression Confession #27}

It's bad enough that I feel alone – it is even worse when those around me don't understand my mental illness.

I have had many co-workers and friends that did not understand why I went through my day intermittently crying or getting frustrated over simple small problems. My friends didn't understand why I cancelled plans constantly or didn't answer their calls.

Eventually people stopped asking me to hang out, they stopped texting or calling...they stopped asking how I was doing.

They would often become silent when I tried to explain that I was depressed or anxious and was struggling that day. People didn't know how to respond. They would try to change the subject or brush off my explanations.

Isolation is common with depression when the depressed person isolates themselves from others...but I think it goes the other way too. Other people don't understand or know how to respond and it isolates the depressed person even more.

Depression is so lonely – and being "shunned" or isolated makes it that much harder.

{Depression Confession #28}

I have nothing to be ashamed of.

I wouldn't be ashamed if I had diabetes and needed to take medication. I wouldn't be ashamed if my appendix ruptured and I needed a hospital stay. I wouldn't be ashamed or embarrassed if I broke my leg and needed physical therapy.

So, I am not ashamed of taking my medication for my brain or needing a hospital stay when I'm suicidal. I am not ashamed for needing to see a therapist once a week. These things help keep me healthy and safe.

Whether I am struggling with a physical ailment or a mental health condition – it doesn't matter. They are ultimately the same thing – something that needs medication/hospitalization or treatment/therapy.

{Depression Confession #29}

Just because you can't see my illness doesn't mean it isn't real.

Depression is one of those invisible illnesses. This means that you cannot see depression or anxiety. You can see a broken bone, you can see the effects of cancer, you can see a wheelchair, and you can see a rash. It makes me sad that people will rush to sign your cast after an accident but will walk away if you tell them you have depression or another invisible illness.

There are actually many invisible illnesses that are not mental health conditions. I'm lucky enough to have multiple invisible illnesses along with my depression. But just because they can't be seen, doesn't mean they are not there.

These aren't made up illnesses to get attention or pity. These are real, diagnosable diseases that affect millions of people. Also – just because you can't see it doesn't make it any less severe than one you can see. My depression can be life-threatening even though people can't see it.

{Depression Confession #30}

When people give me their "advice" on how to "fix" my depression I want to scream.

Everyone has their quick fixes that they love to share. While the intention is great, they are less then helpful.

Here are some of the good ones:

"Have you prayed about it?"

"Just be happy"

"Let it go!"

"If you want to be happy then just do it."

"Just snap out of it."

"You need to get out more."

"You don't look depressed."

"Things aren't that bad – things could always be worse."

"You have to want it."

Yeah...none of these is particularly helpful. You would never say those things to someone who was battling cancer. So why would people think it's okay to say to someone battling depression?

Instead I wish people would say...

"It's okay to not be okay."

"You don't have to go through this alone."

"I'm here to listen."

"What can I do to help you today?"

"You're going to get through this."

"I believe you."

"I'm sorry you are going through this."

These show that a person cares and is listening. This shows the depressed person that they are not being judged – that they have someone in their corner with them.

{Depression Confession #31}

Having depression does not make me weak. Taking medication does not make me weak.

So many think that talking to a therapist or taking medications is a sign of weakness or that something is "wrong" with me. But it is a sign of strength not weakness.

Without the therapy and medications...I would be sick. I may even be dead.

Some people may believe that an anti-depressant is a "band-aid" or a "mask", something that is hiding the real problem underneath. This is not true for those who have true medically diagnosed depression. My depression is a disease caused by an imbalance of chemicals in my brain. I am not hiding behind a mask of anti-depressants – I know my disease and what it takes to live with it. However, I do recognize that there are issues in my past that impact my depression and I face those in therapy.

I am not weak for needing a pill to live. I am strong because I know and accept it. I teach others and try to eliminate the stigma that society has on medication.

The same goes for being hospitalized. At first, I was ashamed that I needed to be hospitalized for my depression and suicidal thoughts. Then I realized that if I had appendicitis, I wouldn't think twice about missing work to get better...it's the same thing! My brain is an organ just as my appendix or heart.

{Depression Confession #32}

You don't have to walk on eggshells around me.

Just because I have depression and suicidal thoughts does not mean you have to treat me with kid gloves or give me special treatment. Mentioning the word suicide or asking me if I'm suicidal is not going to make me kill myself. In fact, it could help save my life. Do not be afraid to ask if someone is suicidal.

Yes, we need to make sure that I am safe and going forward instead of backwards, but walking on eggshells around me just makes me feel belittled. Instead, talk to me like you normally would before the crisis happened.

Getting back to a sense of normalcy is important after a crisis – back into the routine and usual conversations about daily activities and thoughts – not just about the crisis or suicidal thoughts.

Depression Confession Extras:

"People think depression looks like sadness; most the time it does not.

It looks like being called a snob because you work out instead of going out with friends.

It looks like bargaining every morning with yourself just to get out of bed, and sometimes the depression wins. People think you're lazy which feeds your demon.

Depression looks like putting off projects because the thought of failing is too great. The more you put off the worse you feel. People think you're unmotivated because they can't understand the fear.

Many times, depression looks like overachieving because you need to keep proving to yourself, you're good enough because that voice in your head whispers lies. People find you a narcissist or snobby.

Most of all depression looks like loneliness and isolation because your survival tools are constantly misunderstood." – Michelle W.

"I was forced to take medical leave and was told I would be better in a different line of work because of my depression. I have not been able to hold a steady job. People don't take this illness seriously and don't think I'm actually sick because I'm naturally a happy person. I was told I had demons inside me by a group of people who were supposed to be Christians. People don't understand because they can't relate. They think they can relate because they have been sad. They know how incredibly different it is. I think about death almost every day. No one would ever know because no one asks." – Victoria T.

"Both my husband and I take anxiety/depression medication. I have always been very open about my struggles, probably because my family has a long history so it was never something I felt I had to hide. My husband's family are very anti-depression/anxiety medication people, and basically believe it's all in your head. My husband lies to his mom about what his appointments are for and openly tells me he feels ashamed he is on medication which in turn makes me feel like I need to hide my own history from his parents." – Anonymous

"I was diagnosed with depression at a very young age. I stayed the night at my grandparents, and my dad told my grandpa not to forget to give me my anti-depressants to which my grandpa responded, 'What do you have to be depressed about? You are 10!' That was the beginning of me feeling like my emotions were invalid." – Anonymous

"Here's what I wish I knew at fourteen when my next struggle started. You are not "a cry baby". You are not "a drama queen" or "too sensitive". You are not broken or doomed to a painful existence. You have a health condition and your healing can only begin once you start unconditionally loving yourself and calling out the terrible thoughts your depression gives you from your own personality and thoughts. You are a warrior even on the days you don't make it out of bed. Talk about it. Comfort yourself. You deserve it. You're not alone and it does get better. It is not an easy disease to live with but there is treatment and the VAST majority of people feel better with treatment. It may feel hopeless at times; no one medication is right for every person and there are some not so good therapists out there. I've had about 7 over the course of my thirty years. But you will rise up and find strength and resilience you didn't know you had. You can do this. Breathe deep and keep yourself safe." – Kayla V.

"I try really hard not to let people see me or know that I am depressed or my anxiety is taking over. I don't want pity or to be judged." – Jess D.

"People assume my anxiety is self-diagnosed, and I use it as an excuse which my anxiety disorder was diagnosed by a doctor. I never ever use it as an excuse because I don't want to do something. Or people assume I'm mentally weak just because of my depression or anxiety so they assume I can't handle a certain job or tell me to "grow a spine" when I get sad over something." – Aleah D.

Treatment

{Depression Confession #33}

Getting help was the most difficult, terrifying, and BRAVEST thing I've ever done.

I was terrified of being put in the "looney bin". I was terrified of talking about the thoughts in my head. I was terrified of group therapy. I was terrified of medication.

*I was **more** terrified of killing myself than I was of asking for help.*

What did "getting help" look like for me?

The first time, it meant talking to my doctor to get on a new medication. It meant a 3 day stay at an inpatient psychiatric hospital. It meant a 3-week partial hospitalization program and finding a new therapist.

The second time, it meant finding another new therapist and eventually enrolling in another 3-week partial hospitalization program in order to see a psychiatrist to try another new medication.

Being able to see that I was unhealthy and needing help was a huge step. I was denial for so long – but eventually I had to face the facts. I was starting to abuse my medications and drink excessively. It took my husband confronting me to finally "see the light" and get the help I so desperately needed.

{Depression Confession #34}

Talk therapy is an important piece to my treatment.

I didn't want to share my vulnerability to someone that didn't know me. I didn't think that it would be helpful to talk about my day or my troubles.

But come to find out – talking to someone who doesn't know me is quite a release. I'm able to say whatever I feel to someone who has no bias.

Talking through my emotions can be enough to realize what I need to do in my life. My therapist doesn't even have to talk...I eventually come to a place where I know what needs to be done.

Finding a therapist you feel comfortable with is worth the fight.

I have had four different therapists throughout my journey. Some people have more, some people get lucky and find one they connect with right off the bat.

Group therapy was also one of the best therapies during my hospitalization because it allowed me to see that other people are going through the same tough stuff. I was afraid at first but ended up loving it.

Talk therapy in conjunction with medication can often be the best combination for people with depression. It's been the best combination for me. I'm able to get my brain chemistry stabilized while also confronting my distorted thinking and solutions.

{Depression Confession #35}

Hospitalization isn't as scary as it seems.

I was inpatient for 72 hours when I was at my worst depression in 2015. I was terrified of course, but it was the best thing that has happened to me.

Many people are afraid of being "locked up", while yes, it was a locked floor – I still had freedom and was able to see and talk to my family. I was safe and that was the most important thing.

I was released from the hospital to a partial hospitalization program. I came to the hospital 8 AM to 3 PM every week day for approximately three weeks. It was intense talk therapy and medication management with a psychiatrist.

That partial hospitalization program saved my life. Twice.

At the beginning, I was completely against it – I had too much to do, I had to work, I had to make money and be productive.

Then someone asked me, *"What would you do if it was your appendix that was sick, and you needed hospitalization or rehabilitation?"*

I was stunned...it was so obvious at that point!

Of course, I would go to the hospital – I had to get my brain healthy.

{Depression Confession #36}

The journey of finding the right combination of therapy/medication/diet/exercise/self-love can be LONG and extremely difficult. But the key? – KEEP TRYING.

I was on one anti-depressant for most of my teen years and into college. Then it stopped working…. who knew that could happen?!

We then tried many other ones and I struggled with side effects including hallucinations, dizziness, nausea, headaches, and nonexistent libido.

Then I found one that worked! For a while. Then my depression hit another intense low – a mood stabilizer and second anti-depressant were added to my regime.

We are still fine tuning the medications to best fit my depression and anxiety.

I also do talk therapy once or twice a week depending on my needs.

Adding exercise and a healthy/clean diet is also essential to a healthy brain and I am slowly incorporating it back into my life after the relapse of my depression May, 2018.

Self-Care is also important, so I try to make sure that I take time for myself. I read, create art, go for a walk, get my nails done, cuddle my pups, and spend time with my husband and friends.

Finding the right combination of meds, therapy, diet, exercise and self-care can take some time to get right. I still struggle to find a balance but I know that I am on the right track.

Like I said in a previous confession – medication and therapy are a great combination but adding self-care and diet/exercise is also useful in fighting mental illness.

{Depression Confession #37}

I will never miss a dose of my anti-depressant.

I once missed three days of my mood stabilizer and ended up severely suicidal. Even missing one dose can make me feel intense brain fog and dizziness, headaches, or extreme fatigue.

Another time that I forgot to pick up my meds (because I was too depressed to leave the house), I woke up in a fog and with the worst headache. I was irritable, sleepy, and crying about everything. I had panic attacks. I was miserable.

Once back on my meds regularly I am stable!

Lesson Learned – Keep an emergency stock of medication, get them filled at a pharmacy closer to home and NEVER forget to pick your prescriptions.

Remembering to take my medication can be a hassle and I sometimes forget. So, I've started keeping a day's dose in my purse in case I forget before I go to work.

{Depression Confession #38}

My brain without the medication is sick and dangerous.

This is different than the previous confession. When I was first diagnosed with depression and anxiety, I did not want to take medication. I still would prefer to not take medications. But I've come to the realization that my brain needs these medications in order to function correctly. I am okay with that.

I don't fully understand how the brain works but I know the chemicals in my brain are out of whack and my medications bring them back to a stable level where I can function like a normal human being.

I like to compare my brain needing these medications just as a diabetic needs insulin. They are the exact same thing.

So, there should be no shame or embarrassment about taking medications.

{Depression Confession #39}

Self-medicating is common with mental illness.

I turned to alcohol and abusing my prescriptions to deal with the pain and confusion of my depression and anxiety. I'm not proud of this – but it's an important piece of my journey.

I wanted to feel nothing rather than feeling the pain that wouldn't stop. Little did I know – the drinking was just making everything so much worse. I would become suicidal and completely manic. I was out of control.

One night, I drank and drank then got so upset that I took more than double my dose of Xanax. It wasn't that I wanted to die, it was that I wanted it all to go away. I was hospitalized shortly after.

During my hospitalization, I realized how close I was to destroying myself. But with the support of my husband (by getting rid of all the alcohol in our house and controlling the number of drugs I had access to) and my partial hospitalization program, I was able to overcome.

If you are struggling with addiction, please know that there is help. Do not be ashamed and know that it is a sign of strength to reach out.

{Depression Confession #40}

The side effects of my anti-depressants can be horrible – but fighting through them to find a medication that works is SO important.

My mood stabilizer caused me to gain 40 pounds in less than six months, which impacts my self-image and self-confidence. I also have no sex drive whatsoever, which impacts my marriage. I get dizzy to the point of sometimes needing to take a minute for the room to stop spinning which impacts my exercise efforts and daily activities.

Side effects happen to many people taking anti-depressant medications and working with a doctor to determine if the side effects out-weigh the benefits is very important. It's important to follow the doctor's instructions while taking these types of medication as stopping the meds too fast can create with-drawl and dangerous suicidal thoughts (like what I went through as previously described).

Having to choose between the side effects of my anti-depressants like gaining weight or feeling like my depression is finally under some control, really sucks. The balancing act of medications and side effects can be almost impossible. It's a win some, lose some, game of what you can live with and what you can't. But being healthy is the most important.

The weight gain side effect really took its toll, but I remind myself constantly that how I feel is more important than how I look. I would rather have a healthy brain than be down a pant size.

{Depression Confession #41}

Self-care/self-love is NOT selfish.

This is one that I struggle with.

I spend a lot of my time working to help other people both in my career and my volunteer work. I put others first and forget to take care of myself.

I started reminding myself that **I cannot pour from an empty cup.**

I cannot be the person I want to be. I cannot help the people I want to help if I am "empty".

So how do I fill my cup?

I spend time with myself. I go get my nails done. I make art and read books. I love tea, so I will take time to enjoy a cup without being in a hurry or working on something. I also spend time with my dogs and my husband...the simple task of lying on the couch watching television with them fills my cup.

I also go for walks. I try to drink the recommended amount of water and eat as clean as I can. Taking care of your physical being will also benefit your mental health.

Self-care can also be simple things like showering and brushing your hair. Those simple things, let alone the bigger things, can be SO difficult when you're in the depths of depression. But they are so important.

For me – the biggest way I keep my cup filled is saying "No". I was working a full time and a part time job, I was spending every other second working on suicide prevention and mental health advocacy. I was GO GO GOING all the time. I would go weeks without a day "off".

During my second stint with the partial hospitalization program in 2018, I was faced with challenges from my therapists to delete my email app from my phone. I was told to only add one volunteer activity to my calendar per week.

I eventually moved from part-time at one of my jobs to per diem which lowered the days of work I was required to do. I eventually started to delegate other volunteers to attend events and trainings so that I didn't have to go to all of them.

I make sure that I have days off to spend with my husband. I've learned how to balance my work, volunteering, and life. That was my biggest hurdle in finding self-love and I still stumble every once in a while, but I always come back to remind myself to keep my cup full.

{Depression Confession #42}

Medication is not the only form of anti-depressants.

There are many things that can affect mental health. When reading about depression and being overall healthy - diet and exercise are always mentioned. They affect the brain just as much as the rest of the body.

After my first hospitalization I started exercising regularly and felt the best I ever felt... but eventually I stopped and slowly but surely my depression came back. I used to tell everyone that would listen that exercise was the best anti-depressant I found. I still needed my daily medications and therapy, but I saw and felt a change in my life strongly linked to an increase in exercise.

When I eat healthy foods – not only does my body feel good but my brain does too.

Also – being in the sun is a great anti-depressant for me. I don't know about you, but I have a real hard time feeling sad when I'm in the sunshine. I also have one of those fancy lights that help produce the same effects that the sun does to use during the winter.

I also believe that puppies and chocolate are considered anti-depressants, as well as reading a good book.

There are other anti-depressants from holistic options of vitamins and supplements to acupressure/acupuncture and meditation.

Talk to your doctor about additional non-medicinal treatments for depression and anxiety.

Depression Confession Extras:

"I have lived with undiagnosed depression and anxiety since I was a small child. Only recently did I actually get a diagnosis. It wasn't until recently that I decided that it was time to do more than just muddle through it. I was absolutely terrified when I checked into the emergency room where I had only been used to bringing patients to, not being a patient. Being a paramedic, I was so worried that having a mental health history was going to mean losing my license. I had heard once that if you have been hospitalized that you lose your license, or that your employer can terminate you because "you aren't fit for duty." When I checked in, my emotions were all over the place...I was mad because I was in this position. I didn't want any of my co-workers or other hospital staff to know that I was there. I was so worried about what other people were going to think of me and that I would be treated differently. After sitting there for about an hour, I realized that it wasn't about anyone but me! I realized that in order for me to continue to do what I do and love, I had to take care of ME FIRST! For all of my adult life I knew when I needed to bury my emotions and when I could just let myself break down. I got really good at my "public face" and my "private face". As with any illness, it takes a lot of work and learning. I am learning to manage my depression and anxiety and love myself and my life again. The biggest lesson that I have learned from my mental illness is that I AM NOT ALONE AND NEITHER ARE YOU! Keep pushing on because I promise you it will get better!" – Brandon B.

"When I was having depression, it was really hard to go for help. People would think that I was just begging for attention or I was just overthinking it. I was almost to the point of taking my life, and my friend asked if he could help and he has saved my life. I wish people could realize how one person can make a difference. That's all I wish." – Kenny H.

"People always say I seem like the happiest and most bubbly person. I want to feel like those words are true but I knew deep down I am unable to fill those shoes. I've tried medicating. It's a serious trial and error. I've tried 5 different drugs but can't find something to bring me back to the level of "feeling" that used to occur when I was younger. I had serious body dysmorphia when I first acknowledged my depression. I distinctly remember eating only 1 peach for an entire day before realizing that I had a problem. Depression comes in waves and, even though it's come so far, I still wish it wasn't as stigmatized because it's a true issue in my life and many others." – Megan H.

"For as long as I can remember I have struggled with anxiety, depression and suicidal ideations. Going on prescription medication for the first time when I was in college, I hated how I felt. I tried multiple different medications, some with nasty side effects, some helped...most did not. I finally found one that helped with minimal side effects but taking it made me feel like a failure, that regardless of how much therapy I did I could not help myself without pills.

After losing my Aunt to suicide last winter, I debated going back on anti-depressants. The aunt I lost was the one who had talked me into getting help before and I found myself constantly wondering...'Why am I still here when she isn't?' I felt like I had to be okay because she wasn't. But really, I haven't been okay for quite some time and that was completely unrelated to her. I still feel like there must be reason that I am here...a reason why she is not...and I know I will probably never learn that reason, but I have HOPE that the reason is a dang good one.

This past week, I finally called my doctor and she prescribed the medication that I had been on, gone off, gone back on and gone off over the last decade. Today I took the first pill. Instead of feeling the shame and guilt for not being okay enough to do things on my own, for the first time I feel like I am STRONG...strong enough to realize that my mental health is just as important as my physical health and it is GOOD to take something that will help me to be healthy." – Angela P.

"Many days I feel like I'm a burden and bothersome. I feel like I am a burden to my therapist. Most days I feel like doing what's best for my health is a wasting/taking up someone else's time who needs the therapist more than me and like it's pointless for me to go." – Heather M

Recovery

{Depression Confession #43}

Recovery is not linear. It's full of ups and downs and more ups and downs with some backwards and sideways thrown in.

What I mean is that if you think of the journey of depression as a line of peaks and valleys – each episode of depression (valley) is less steep and dangerous than the one previously. Even having ups and downs my trend of recovery is still heading upwards.

It's almost like two steps forward, one step back type of journey. It is extremely frustrating. One day I feel great and think I'm getting the handle on my life again, and then, boom, the next day I can't get out of bed. Which leads to distorted thinking such as, "I'm a failure" or "I can't do anything right." But in reality, if I looked at how far I have come, I can see that I am not a failure and I'm obviously doing something right considering I'm healthier than before.

It's important to realize that there will be ups and downs and that is okay. That is part of the recovery.

{Depression Confession #44}

Feeling happiness for the first time in months is like finally seeing the world in color after it being black and white for so long.

To be honest feeling genuine happiness after so long of feeling miserable is almost like being high on life. It feels like I can breathe after being underwater for too long. It feels like a weight has been lifted off of my shoulders and I can finally see the colors of the world without the film of pain and darkness.

I also learned how to answer some of the questions that constantly haunted me:

- Why am I crying? – Because you care, because you were hurt. It's okay to cry.
- Why do I care so much? – Because you're a good person who has empathy.
- Why do I hurt so much? – Because you've had heartbreak and that's okay to feel to hurt.
- Why me? – Because I'm one in four who struggle with mental illness.
- Why do I have to go through this? – Because it's making me a better person who can help others going through similar things.
- Why can't people understand? – Because no one has taught them, and because they don't have depression.
- Why don't people even try? – Because they're scared of something they don't understand.
- Why do they leave? – Again...because they're scared of what they don't understand.

- Why can't I be happy? – Because I suffer from depression and that makes it difficult...**but not impossible.**

{Depression Confession #45}

Just because I am in recovery does NOT mean I'm immune to bad days.

It's important to know that bad days will happen to everyone. But for those of us who live with depression, even those on medication and seeing a therapist - the bad days can tear us apart.

These bad days are extremely difficult because it feels like I've failed for that day...that every day is going to be bad now. That is untrue. A bad day is not indicative of a relapse. A bad day is just that – a bad day. Now a string of bad days or having more bad days than good days could be a sign of my depression deepening.

I always say that if you can find one thing to make you smile each day – then that day was worth living. So, on the days that I can't smile...I make sure I watch some type of comedy show so that I get a laugh or two in that day. (My go to favorite is Big Bang Theory or the movie Pitch Perfect.)

Even on hard days – I know that there are better ones coming.

{Depression Confession #46}

Relapse can happen.

I have relapsed multiple times after my initial hospitalization. The first major relapse I had, I was able to get it under control myself. But the second most recent relapse is the one that I'm still fighting with the help of different medications, a new therapist and psychiatrist. This second relapse has taken its toll. I thought I was never going to get through it (while I'm still in the journey of recovering from this relapse, the worst is over).

But this step back does not take away what I have achieved. I look back at the journey I've already made and know that I can get through this again.

I often express the sentiment that, "it isn't fair...I don't understand why I have to keep going through this". Isn't once in hell enough? Let alone twice or more.

But through the storm...through the darkness, I always learn something new about myself.

{Depression Confession #47}

Sometimes relapse comes before I even know what happened.

It comes in slow motion and sneaks up from the shadows – it is little things at first. A bad day here, a bad day there, some extra anxiety, some sleeping in and taking extra naps...and then BOOM – it's right in my face, full blown depression once again. It turns my good days to dust and my laughter to tears. It puts my smile to sleep.

How did I not see it?
When did this happen?
Did anyone else notice?

I feel like I failed, like I let the depression get the best of me once more. It makes asking for help (again) even harder...I should have been better. Who is going to believe me now? Who will still support me through another round of this war? Will anyone listen?

This has happened to me a few times now through this journey. Where one day, I wake up and realize I've been falling into depression all along.

I try to be aware of my emotions as much as I can in order to keep track of my depression and its early signs that can be missed. I've made lists of what to "look out for", including sleeping too much, always being tired, an increase in anxiety, irritability, and crying without really knowing why. They are similar to my safety plan warning signs. It's important to pick up the signs earlier in order to stop them before they get dangerous.

{Depression Confession #48}

Recovery doesn't happen overnight.

I wish I could say that my recovery was fast and beautiful. But it hasn't been. It's been long and difficult. Depression isn't "cured" just because you take a pill or see a therapist. It isn't "cured" just because you want it to be.

This has probably been one of the hardest things for me to grasp. I just want to be better NOW. Those who know me know that I am not a very patient person.

I don't want to have to work for recovery – I just want it to be. Wishful thinking, I suppose, because you have to work for it. You have to take the steps needed to reach recovery.

This isn't easy. This is a mission of hard work and making small progresses each day. There are setbacks, but with perseverance, I will overcome them. Recognizing that recovery doesn't happen overnight or even in a couple days was a big revelation to me. It meant that I had to take it seriously and fight back. Once I came to terms that I had a fight ahead of me, I was able to take back control of my brain and my life.

{Depression Confession #49}

I am worthy of recovery.

I used to think that recovery was a far-fetched aspiration and I would never achieve it. I believed that I was never going to get better and that this pain would ultimately lead me to taking my life. I believed it would be like this forever...the unbearable pain and darkness. I believed that I wasn't even worthy of recovery. That is one of those sneaky little lies that my brain was telling me.

Because, I am worthy of recovery. In fact, I am worthy of a smile and laughter. I am worthy of my future. I am worthy of a family who understands. I am worthy of a recovery that brings me back to life.

I am worthy.

&& so are you.

Depression Confession Extras:

"There comes a time with depression where one day you wake up and suddenly everything feels wrong. You feel physically ill getting out of bed feels like you are trying to stand with a hundred-pound weight on your shoulder. You know you have to get up and go to work or school but it doesn't matter. You just want to lay there and watch the world pass you by blessedly without you interacting in it.

I have felt this several times in my life. Sometimes I overcame. And I slowly stand up on my own two feet and take the first few steps of the day. I endure. Other times I don't overcome. I drown. And that's ok too. You can't win all the time or there would be no glory when you actually do win. Beating back the depression, even temporarily, is one of the greatest victories you can have. No one will ever know the struggle you go through, or how much of a hero you are. But you will. And in your darkest times you can reflect on that, and draw strength." – Cody S.

"Recovery does not happen in the blink of an eye, but sometimes it takes major life changes to get there. Removing toxic people. Changing jobs. Changing homes. Changing partners. Realizing the things that are contributing to your anxiety and depression and being strong enough to change that all while trying to "fix" yourself." – Bridgette B.

"I wish people would understand that this is a chronic illness – it isn't just going to go away. Just because I'm not crying everyday anymore or having panic attacks doesn't mean I'm not anxious or depressed. It just means that I've taken a step forward – but I still have a lot of steps to go." – Anonymous

"I wish people would know that I don't get to decide when and how my depression will hit me. That sometimes it's like lightning and never strikes twice in the same spot. I wish people knew and understood that when I am severely depressed, I'm not trying to bring the mood down. I'm keeping to myself and being quiet to do the least amount of damage possible to the situation. I wish people knew that depression isn't some jacket you can shrug out of if the weather changes. It's more like a huge complicated winter coat and you want to take it off. But you can't find the zipper because you are wearing three pairs of gloves and there are 30-pound weights attached to your wrists." – Cody S.

"Sometimes I don't believe that I will ever "recover" from my depression. Even though I have more good days than bad days I still know that my depression is there in the background. I hope to someday recover fully, but I know it's a fight and not a short one." – Anonymous

"The hardest thing I have learned with my recovery with borderline personality disorder, depression and anxiety is that it's called recovery and not recovered because it takes time. And as in time it can take years. And while still in recovery, there are days that it takes minutes to get me to the next. I was very surprised going into recovery in the past year that it wasn't what I thought. It's not all sparkle and rainbows, and it's still a lot of dark and a lot of tears. No two recoveries are the same dealing with mental health!" – Jen G

"Recovery is transitional and goes back and forth. Just when you think you are doing well, sometimes it doesn't take much to push you back down the dark alley you were in (and thought you had escaped). But recovery takes work, concentration and a commitment to not allow yourself to be pushed back down the dark alley. When it is happening, take control and just realize, you have taken control and can do it again. Seek your higher power to walk with you out of the darkness where you are being pushed. Be positive. Know you can do it. Regain your positive control and don't look anywhere but to the light! Six years and I still have bumps in the road - but each time - I look to the light and am thankful for all which is good! Few know of my darkness when it still happens. I hide it well some say. The deepness of depression isn't something always seen by your family and friends. Please don't be afraid to tell them. It is time for a hug!" – Lois H.

Supporting a Loved One

{Depression Confession #50}

Loving someone with anxiety or depression can be frustrating.

My husband struggles with severe anxiety and even though I struggle with anxiety myself, it is difficult and frustrating to see him fighting so hard.

His anxiety interferes with his daily activities including his job, driving, our marriage, and social interactions. I often get frustrated when we are going someplace that should be fun, but he gets anxious and doesn't want to go.

I try to understand and help him through his anxiety, but sometimes I let my frustration show and can get angry/upset with him. It's normal to be frustrated. I mean, I get frustrated with myself when my own anxiety interferes with life. I know he gets frustrated with me when my anxiety gets in the way.

But in reality – I know it is not his fault. He can't control the anxiety any more than I can. It is his brain that is lying to him and making him freak out...the best thing I have found that I can do is just be there. He doesn't need me to say anything – just be there.

So even when it's frustrating and hard, I try my best to just be there for him and remind him that this will pass, and it'll all be okay.

{Depression Confession #51}

Watching someone I love struggle with mental illness is heartbreaking.

Watching my husband fight his anxiety is so hard. I just want to take his pain and worries away. I don't want him to suffer what I suffer from. It breaks my heart to see him when he is in distress.

I also have a close-knit group of friends who have all been impacted by suicide in some way. Many of them also struggle with depression and suicidal thoughts. I always let them know that I am there for them no matter the time or place.

I have taken a friend to the hospital for a psychological evaluation for feeling suicidal. I have visited multiple friends in the inpatient hospitalization program. I have referred friends to services and resources in our community. I have sat with them and cried with them. Each time, my heart hurts so much for them – I know the pain they are feeling and I wouldn't wish it on my worst enemy let alone a best friend.

I watched my dad as he struggled after overdosing a few months before his suicide. I watched him fight his demons although I didn't quite understand how much trouble he was in.

It is not easy to see your friends or your family fighting to stay alive.

But like I've learned with my husband's struggle with anxiety, I often find that being there and not saying anything is what they need the most. Someone to listen to them without interrupting. Someone who lets them know it's okay to not be okay and that asking for help is a sign of strength not weakness.

{Depression Confession #52}

Supporting a loved one is not easy but is so important.

It can be very hard to support a loved one who struggles with mental illness. It can be especially difficult when the loved one is pushing you away or is in denial of their illness.

But here are some key things I do to support my loved ones.

- Listen to them non-judgmentally. Let them share their struggles on their own terms.

- Remind them that it's okay to seek help – that it's a sign of strength and growth.

- Be there for them. Whether that means being with them at home or taking them to get help.

- Check in on them from time to time – even if you think they are doing well...just check on them with a simple text message or phone call.

- Remember that it's not their fault that they get so anxious they can't leave the house and they cancel plans...try to come up with plans that they find do-able.

But most of all – *remind them that you love them unconditionally.*

{Depression Confession #53}

When it's me struggling, I need support - not fixing.

Accept me and love me instead of trying to fix the problem or cure me. The power of just being there is enough. Accept that this is part of our relationship.

Most of the time I know what I need to do to make myself feel better but I don't have energy or willpower to do it. You can help me – pour me a cup of tea, put on my favorite funny TV show, get my fuzzy blanket, buy me my favorite treat…but you don't have to try to "fix" me. Give me reminders and encouragement that I will get through this and that it'll be okay.

I don't need someone telling me that I "need" to get outside or that I "have to" do something to make my depression better. I need gentle reminders that going for a walk or going out to dinner is good for me.

I may be broken and I may need your help to put me back together but don't force it.

Sit with me if I'm quiet. Listen to me if I'm talking. Hold my hand if I'm crying. Hug me if I'm struggling. Be there with me.

{Depression Confession #54}

Hope is healing.

Hope. It is the glue that holds me together.

When my depression is at its worst – I find that hope is the light to drive out its darkness. It's the hope that tomorrow will be better – that the storm will pass.

When others struggle, I try to give them the same hope and love that I hold dearly. Showing others that there is hope and love in this world no matter what they are facing is pivotal to supporting them in their fight.

Depression has a nasty habit of taking hope away – but with the help of those around me, we are able to uncover the hope, healing and love needed to overcome depression.

Depression Confession Extras:

"The worry, the worry, the worry! When the phone rings, is it a happy call, an angry call, a scared crying call, is it a panic attack? I'm afraid to pick up the phone never knowing what is waiting for me on the other end. My heart drops to my stomach with worry when my phone rings. I take a deep breath and answer with a smile. Most of the time it's nothing.

The mood swings. One minute they are laughing with you, the next they are angry, mad and yelling. What did I do? It does not take much to set them off, could be the tiniest of things. It could be something I did, someone else did, or no one did anything. Maybe it was the movie we were watching. On the way home from work I have the constant wonder – what is the mood at home? Is it a good day or a bad day? You learn to roll with it.

Forget about having a relaxed dinner and a movie, a trip to the grocery store, visiting a friend, or even a holiday gathering. They don't want to go and I make the decision to go without them. There is nothing relaxing about "getting" out. The constant worry about them the whole time, what are they doing? Are they sad? Are they mad I went without them? Are they going to fix themselves something to eat, are they drinking or maybe they are doing fine and it's none of these? Then there are the phone calls – how much longer are you going to be? How long is the movie? Are you eating while you are out? What am I going to eat? Are you on your way home yet?

Then there is the guilt for leaving them home alone. I should be there with them, fixing them food, making sure they are okay, making sure they are taking their meds or taking the correct dosages and just being there if they need me. Then there is the guilt of just having a good time.

The hardest thing to do is to take your loved one to the hospital for help with their mental health crisis. The first step is getting in the door. No matter how hard or how much you want to help them yourself, the best thing is to get them the proper care. I cry all the way home after leaving them or visiting them. It is so hard to see your loved one suffer. They are getting the care they need, they cannot harm themselves, and knowing they are on the mend, eases and settles the mind. I preach to them the same things I tell myself – stay strong, you are doing the right thing." – Stacy P.

"The biggest lesson I've learned by loving someone with severe mental health issues is to never lose focus on yourself. Allowing yourself to walk away, even if it's only temporary, in order to maintain your own sanity is okay. And never, ever hesitate to call professionals when you can no longer safely handle the situation." – Meghan B.

"My boyfriend; we have been together a year and a half and he's had depression the whole time. He isn't the best version of himself and hasn't been since I met him about 2.5 years ago. We continually go around and round because I, not being depressed now but have been a on and off, try to get him to partake in things that make him happy or try to encourage positive habits that could help. He can't wrap his mind around any of these things. It never alters the way he loves and cares for me, but it holds him back immensely. He has no sense of time management, no drive or motivation to do simple tasks, and his body aches constantly. He's always dreaming of different things for his life but never actually tries to obtain those goals. I have researched online and through books the best ways to help and encourage him while not seeming like "I'm stressing him out" (his words) as well as trying to help him through things he genuinely enjoys. But it never seems like enough. Don't get me wrong we have many good days, but the bad days are bad sometimes and it's hard to stand on the sidelines and watch the person you love struggle so badly.

My Father; This one hits a lot closer to home. For as long as I can remember vivid memories of my dad, he's never been 'happy'. We never were particularly close. He's always shown me in a million other ways he loves me and will always provide for me, but we've never talked about feelings, never really kissed or hugged, and until recently barely even said 'I love you'. As someone looking from the outside, I could sense that my dad wasn't happy but you never really know until you hear it firsthand. This summer we attended a baseball game and he spilled the entire beans to me. That for YEARS, he hasn't been happy. He told me straight to my face that he loves my mom, sister, I, the dogs, blah, blah, blah, but he's not happy. To know that your dad loves you, but isn't happy about anything in his life is hard.

He told me nothing makes him happy. The two dogs he bought, the family he started, the $300,000 house he built us and the pole barn he just recently had built as well as filled with boy toys. He constantly struggles and refuses to ask for help or even speak out to us to how we could potentially help him. He refuses to seek help. He refuses to do anything. As morbid as this sounds, sometimes I think that someday I'll come home and be the one to find him. I'm sorry that's so morbid but to know that he's so unhappy and not knowing an ounce what to do. I cry.

Both these men mean an absolute ton to me but I struggle daily to be someone they need. To be some ray of sunlight. And to hopefully make them feel better. I will continue to educate myself and listen to them so I can be the best version of myself for them." – Ally D.

"I wish people could understand that just because I look like I have my life together from the outside...makeup done, hair done, thriving at work, hitting the gym, I'm literally dying inside. This is all me fighting for my life. I need them to reach out and support me in this battle for my life. The biggest thing you can do is let someone know that you are there for them. Ask them if they are still okay, and what you can do to help. They may not have the energy to ask for it. Don't assume that just because outside appearances show that I am okay, doesn't mean I am. Feeling alone in the battle seems so overwhelming, but reaching out seems overwhelming. Just ask that friend that "seems okay" if they are really okay." – Anonymous

"My friend Brooke didn't have an easy home life. The man her mother was dating at the time was very mentally abusive. Through all this abuse, Brooke went into a deep depression. Self-harming, wishing she was dead, thinking nobody loved her. One night we finally convinced her parents to let her stay the night at my house. Everything was going great...until everybody went to sleep. I woke up because I had to use the bathroom. I opened the door to the bathroom and found Brooke had cut herself multiple times on her thighs. She was crying, I started crying. She begged and begged me not to go get my mom. So, I didn't. I cleaned her up and we went back to bed. At that time, I thought I was being a good friend by not telling my mom. However, Brooke's home life didn't get any better. Her mom's boyfriend just got more abusive. So, she ended up coming to live with us. Brooke's life got much better at my house. Until the weekend her parents asked her to just come stay for the weekend. I got a call saying that she tried to kill herself and they were taking her to the hospital. She went to a mental facility after that for a few weeks. I went to see her. Her parents never came to see her. When she got out, she went to live with her grandma, away from her parents. She ended up getting a degree and has a child and lives a full and good life now. Brooke messaged me a while back saying thank you. Thank you that my family and I supported her and saved her life. I may not be able to help the entire world, but I'm going to try, one person at a time. I just want people to know that even if you have depression, people still care and you can conquer it and live the life you love." - Anonymous

"Nobody quite realizes how terrifying it is to parent a child with depression and mental health issues. How hard it is every single day to make sure she isn't going to hurt herself. How it is to get that call that she's in the hospital after another suicide attempt. The sleepless nights of staying up on suicide watch with her all night because she's had a bad day. How frustrating it is to know you cannot protect her from all the bad things in the world, teach her all about bad people and how to be safe, but not know how to protect her from herself. How hard it is to not be able to take her pain away, wishing you could take that pain on yourself. The feeling of wanting to "fix" it, but having no idea how. What it's like to be the mother of a child who is manic depressive and has borderline personality disorder. The fear that I have every second, of every day, that it could be her last day. The last "I love you". The last "good night". The last hug. The last everything." – Bridgette B.

"I am losing the love of my life and our marriage as a result of depression. My husband and I have always had depression struggles but have never been strong enough to get help. We would both lock everything so deep inside until this would become unbearable. My husband attempted suicide before getting to a place where he felt he could ask for help. But this came at a cost. He was filled with so much grief, sadness and guilt that he had misplaced and, in an attempt to make sense of it all, he began to blame me. Suddenly, like a switch, he had decided that I was the cause of all of his depression and by getting away from me, he could find himself and be happy.

So, after eleven years of love and eleven years of things left unsaid, he threw in the towel. All of his grief swiftly turned to anger and hatred towards me and yet, I still have no answer as to where this came from. A month ago, he was my loving husband sending me poetry, kissing me and laughing with me. Literally over night, I became his worst enemy. I am trying so desperately to unearth any answers and save our marriage because, underneath everything, I know he's there. It's been an incredible struggle for me to watch him go through this. I have no hatred for what he has become, only hope that he may return. I know that all I can do is get help for myself and just hold on for now. Despite everything, I want him to understand that I am here for him, I love him. Depression is so much more than hard times in your relationship. It is enveloping and it morphs and distorts even the most beautiful parts of life until they are suddenly unrecognizable. "– Anonymous

Surviving a Suicide Loss

{Depression Confession #55}

A death by suicide is very different than a death by any other means.

Death is never an easy thing whether it's from an accident, a physical illness or a suicide. However, a loss by suicide has some differences.

While there are always questions of "Why them?" and "Why did this happen?", these questions are much more loaded for those who have lost someone to suicide.

There is a high level of guilt. There are many questions that we loss survivors ask, such as, "What could I have done?", "What if I would have said something or did something different?", and "How could I have missed the signs?"

After losing my dad, I was faced with these questions. I was riddled with guilt as I wish I would have said something the last time I saw him. Guilt that I don't even remember the last words he said to me.

Guilt is a common emotion felt with the loss of someone to suicide. It's one that many survivors must work through. It took me a long time, but I now know that my father's death was not my fault...there was nothing more that I could have done. While it's not an easy concept to come to terms with, it gave me a sense of freedom after all, that it wasn't me that caused his death, it was his illness.

{Depression Confession #56}

Grieving is not linear.

Healing from a suicide loss, or any loss for that matter is not linear. There is no "one path" one must take to heal from grief.

There are the five stages of grief: denial, anger, bargaining, depression and acceptance. Most people are familiar with those steps. What a lot people don't realize is that these stages don't have to go in order. The stages can end then come back. They can last for months or years after the loss.

For me, I was in denial and bargaining for a few months. Then I hit depression and acceptance. It wasn't until a couple years after the loss of my dad that I hit anger and then started the process over again with denial then depression and finally acceptance.

Everybody's journey with healing is different, just as everyone's journey with mental illness is different. It's important to know that it's okay to go back and forth and hit the stages of grief more than once. In fact, it's completely normal.

{Depression Confession #57}

There is no right or wrong way to grieve.

Just as the stages of grief may not occur in order, there is no right or wrong way to grieve.

Some people may choose to attend support groups to help heal while others do not. Some people may choose to go through therapy for help and some do not.

Members of the same family can grieve very differently. Some may decide they want to talk about the loss, or they may not want to talk about the person who passed at all. Others may want to talk about the loss frequently, as they want to remember the person they've lost.

I chose to make suicide prevention my mission. I decided to organize a walk, in memory of my dad. That was my way of grieving. I chose to face his suicide and turn our tragedy into something positive.

{Depression Confession #58}

I am not ashamed of my father's suicide.

My dad fought depression and chronic physical pain. He was sick – he had a disease that was relentless. My dad was brave, and he was strong. He fought for months, maybe even years, before depression took him Dec. 22nd, 2010.

It would be easy to blame him for the pain my family has endured. It would be easy to be angry. In fact, I've felt both of those things. The one thing I never did was be embarrassed or ashamed. I wouldn't be ashamed if he had died in a car accident or if he died from heart attack so why would I feel ashamed that he died from depression?

I am actually proud of him for fighting so long and so hard. It must have been extremely painful for him. I know it must have been painful because I have been there – I have been suicidal and I know that it's excruciating and nothing makes sense.

My dad was sick and the treatments just weren't working. His depression became life threatening and ultimately fatal.

I am not ashamed of him or his death. I am proud to be his daughter.

{Depression Confession #59}

Suicide is not selfish.

One of the biggest things I hate to hear when people talk about death by suicide is that the person was being selfish or that they weren't thinking of anything but themselves.

This is false.

A brain that is fighting suicidal thoughts is sick. It forms a type of tunnel vision where they can't see another way out. The brain lies and says that their families will be better off without them.

I know this because I have been there – I have felt the suicidal impulses. I've also felt the pain of being left behind after a suicide of a loved one. But that knowledge did not stop my suicidal thoughts. In fact it made my battle that much worse because I felt like I was failing my family.

My dad was not selfish – he spent his life helping others by being a volunteer firefighter and EMS. He was in the military fighting for our country. He was far from selfish. He was sick.

Dying by suicide is not selfish – it's the end result of a fatal mental illness.

{Depression Confession #60}

My father's suicide changed me.

I was a freshman in college when my dad died. I was getting used to all that dorm life had to offer and my grades reflected that. I was staying at college on the weekends because I didn't want to go home.

But that Christmas break – everything changed. My dad died, and I knew I had to be better. So, I pushed myself and got all A's that next semester. I started looking for ways to bring a positive to my dad's death. I found it in the summer of 2011.

I attended my first Out of the Darkness walk with The American Foundation for Suicide Prevention (AFSP). It started an amazing journey of finding healing and hope. Then I organized a walk in my hometown and eventually moved it to Lansing, MI. That walk has now raised over $100,000 for suicide prevention programs and research along with survivor of suicide loss resources.

I have journeyed to Washington D.C. with the AFSP to advocate for mental health reform and funding for suicide prevention. I helped organize International Survivors of Suicide Loss Days. I've gone to schools, businesses and health fairs to share our resources, programs and trainings.

My entire life has been altered because of my dad's suicide. I choose to turn my family's heartbreaking tragedy into something positive so that others would never have to go through what we did.

But his suicide changed me in another way...

My own mental illness was starting to get the best of me. I would say, "If my dad died this way – then I could too. That I probably would." My depression deepened, and I started to spiral. It was with the help of my family and my husband that I was able to get the help I needed. I know now, that just because my dad died by suicide does not mean that I will too. Yes, my risk is higher, but nothing is concrete.

I've spent the last 10 years of my life fighting my mental illness in various forms and at various times just like my dad. My dad's death has given me strength and with that strength, I will continue fighting my depression and anxiety. I will continue to be a mental health advocate and I will always stay.

Depression Confession Extras:

"It's been 10 years since my fiancé died by suicide. I'm the one that found him, and I can't bear to see suicides on tv or movies and I can anticipate them happening. I have to close my eyes. I don't know if that will ever go away. I also suffer from PTSD from his suicide. For the first year after he passed, I had to get on an anti-depressant to cope with life." – Tressa S.

"Some time ago, I was forced into a divorce from the mother of my children, shortly after I started adjusting to that new life, I lost my brother to his own demons. I suppose this is where my own demons started growing. Today I find myself dependent upon others for motivation. For happiness I seek out others to fill voids in my life. Seeking others for my happiness has led me to bad decisions in life, love and finance. Momentarily, I can find joy in life, but then the reality of the situation becomes clear. I fall back to emptiness and loneliness that can be overwhelming at times. The spark to solve the emptiness is ever elusive for me…some days I find it in work. Other times in communication with family. Sometimes the search goes on for weeks until I find something that engrossed my mind so deeply, I forget about the things holding me down…until the next time and it all starts again." – Larry P.

"January 10th, 1986, is a day that changed our lives forever. My mom had an appointment to find out if she was pregnant for me, unfortunately that did not happen. Her oldest brother fought a hard battle with depression, and he took his life. Fast forward, September 1986, I was born. I was his name sake. I was the piece they held on to. While I never met my uncle, I feel as though I grew up with him. I've heard many stories through the years about what he was like, and who he was. He left a natural hole for everyone in our family, and ironically, one for me too! I feel his presence through my mom, my grandma, and his only child, who is my cousin Sarah. We celebrate my uncle through each holiday. His memory is still alive in each and every one of us. Suicide isn't something that just affects those present in the moment. It's an event that ripples through the family for many years leaving a lasting effect on each person differently." – Danielle G.

"Life after losing someone to suicide was like living in a fog and cold darkness. I started to see that I didn't know if I was coming or going. When I couldn't remember what I wore the day of her funeral services I realized I was in trouble. The entire outfit vanished and I never got memory of what had happened. I also found myself so confused in time and dates. It seemed like those days collided and then the world kept on living while I died inside. Wanting desperately to be close to her, I would go and lay on her graveside till the groundskeeper would tell me they were fixing to lock up. I wanted so desperately to be with her. As I cried, I remember begging the time to rewind and let me step in and save her. Life has and never will be the same, but I had to fight to live though I'm broken inside because I had family and they couldn't see I was losing myself. Finding AFSP was the key to hope, the will for my fight, and the way to make a difference in her memory. Though life will never be the same, I go forward in hopes to touch or save someone's life by advocating, educating and being present to listen." – Annette B.

"This coming February is the five-year anniversary of losing my 16-year old brother to suicide. I always thought that would be my fate. Being six years older than my brother, he watched me as I spiraled out of control when I was 16 and harmed myself for years to come after that. It was so obvious that I was hurting, as I had numerous breakdowns a day and cried all the time. My brother never showed us any signs he was hurting. He was the funny one, the brave one the hardworking one. So, when I got the call from my mom that he died, I assumed he got in a car accident as the roads were absolutely covered in ice and snow when my roommate drove me home. When I arrived home, my mom said he killed himself. My legs completely gave out from under me. 'My brother? Are you sure it was him?' To this day, I have a small part of me that believes he is still out there. No, not in heaven, but that he just moved away and will be back someday. When he comes walking in the door, I will slap him on the head for missing out on all of these important moments I have had to handle on my own since then. Being an only child again is something I never bargained for, and something I might never fully accept. I am lucky though, a few months before he died, I wrote him a letter telling him why my parents adopting him was the best thing that ever happened to me. I got to read that letter at his funeral in front of almost a thousand people. I know he knew full well how much he meant to me, but I will eventually have to forgive myself that love isn't always enough to keep people here. I miss him every second of every day. To be perfectly honest, it isn't any easier for me now. I've just become better at pretending. As the holidays approach this year, I am reminded once again of my immense sadness amidst what seems like the joy of everyone else. I have learned throughout these past five years that I am not alone in this feeling, but that so many others have become good at pretending as well. If you are reading this and relate at all, just know you are not alone in your sadness." – Anonymous

Closing Confession

When I started this book – I figured that no one would be very interested and that I was writing it more for myself. But once I asked for others to submit their confessions...my eyes were opened. It still shocks me to know that so many people, just in my network, are affected by suicide or mental illness.

This book started out as just my story with depression. Now, it includes the stories of over 50 other people who have been impacted by mental illness.

This book is so much more than a collection of depression confessions. When 1 in 4 people are affected by mental illness these confessions are reality for so many.

Everyone's journey is different, no one story is the same as the next. I feel it is important to share our stories in order to empower others to do the same. So, it is my hope, that this book starts a conversation, breaks the stigma, gives hope and understanding and allows others to know that they are not alone.

Thank You

There are so many people that need to be thanked for pushing me, for guiding me and for loving me.

Thank you to the wonderful people who helped make this book possible by sharing their stories, journeys and confessions.

Thank you, Mike, for being the amazing husband that you are. Thank you for supporting me in all I do, for being my rock, and for being my sunshine when depression takes me into its depths. Thank you for loving me through this and for always making me smile through the rainstorms.

Thank you to my mom and sister for always being there to talk to or simply spend time with me when I can't be alone. Thank you for working to understand depression and loving me.

Thank you to my AFSP family – it's because of you that I am still alive and fighting for mental health advocacy and suicide prevention. Our fight is not easy but together we are stronger.

Thank you to my co-workers who support me in my journey to heal and grow. I honestly don't know where I would be without the love and support that you have shown me in the past year.

Thank you to my therapist for pushing me to do my best and for helping me set boundaries in my life in order to keep my mental health in check.

Thank you to my dogs Zeus and Gordie for always letting me squeeze and love you.

Made in the USA
Middletown, DE
10 August 2019